carrier

**UNTANGLING
THE
DANGER
IN MY DNA**

BONNIE J. ROUGH

COUNTERPOINT
BERKELEY

Author's Note: This is a memoir about my family, and it includes stories, scenes,
and voices from the generations before mine. To piece together this history, I used
interviews, photographs, letters, documents, artifacts, site visits, and my intuition.
I undertook this project in a search for the truth—my family's and my own. Since
detailed research could take me only so far into long-lost incidents and sentiments,
I used disciplined imagination to re-create conversations and details—but without
embellishment or pure invention. My abiding intention has been to tell a true
story, in the way I understand it.

Library of Congress Cataloging-in-Publication Data

Rough, Bonnie J.
    Carrier : untangling the danger in my DNA / by Bonnie J. Rough.
        p. cm.
    ISBN-13: 978-1-58243-578-7
    ISBN-10: 1-58243-578-2
    1. Rough, Bonnie J.—Health. 2. Ectodermal dysplasia—Patients—Biography. I.
Title.

RL793.R68 2010
362.198'30092—dc22
[B]

                        2009052553

Cover design by Natalya Balnova
Interior design by Elyse Strongin, Neuwirth & Associates, Inc.

Printed in the United States of America

COUNTERPOINT
2117 Fourth Street
Suite D
Berkeley, CA 94710

www.counterpointpress.com

Distributed by Publishers Group West

10 9 8 7 6 5 4 3 2 1

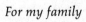

For my family

prologue

It began with a burst of sunshine, a bad taste in the air, a hiccup as one cell tried to transfer its data to another. It began long before me, your mother. A genetic disorder, carried invisibly by mothers and passed to sons, snakes through our family tree. It is a fragment of history we can trace, a tiny bundle of stories floating in our blood.

The primary symptoms of your condition are sparse hair, peg- or cone-shaped teeth, and the inability to sweat. At every moment, a normal human body engages in a struggle against death by heat or cold. A person with sweat glands fights overheating with perspiration. But a body without sweat glands flies on faith, staving off death without the checks and balances of normal human physiology.

The secondary symptoms include distinctive facial features, such as dark circles around the eyes and a saddle-nose deformity: a deep depression where the bridge of the nose should be. Sufferers have trouble breathing, so they have trouble sleeping, and so they have trouble keeping awake. Because of their tired appearance and sallow skin, they often appear ill, even when they feel fine. On the other hand, many often are ill. Immunodeficiency associated with the condition may lead to a lifetime of infections. All this leads others to view sufferers of this disorder as weak, incompetent, possessed of problems.

It is called hypohidrotic ectodermal dysplasia, or HED. The

older a man with this disorder gets, the more trouble he may have getting his body to respond to medication. The more exhausted he may become, the worse for his self-esteem. Despite the fact that HED is said not to limit life expectancy, I have learned this: The more pain a sufferer feels, the more he may wish to die.

As I tell you these stories, you are nothing but a phantom. You are a strange presence, a spirit somehow alive. By turns I feel compelled to greet you, to apologize to you, to nurture you, and to frighten you away. You have taken up a place in my heart. Before long, you might take up a place in my womb. We could find ourselves thus: you, a fetus, with a skull the size of a cherry and a wisp of body trailing. Me, and your father, deciding whether to bring you into the world.

Soon after our wedding, you came into my dreams: a blond-haired baby boy, with a round face and little spectacles bespeaking your strange intelligence. We walked on the shore. We lay in the sand. The air blew wet and salty. You told me to look for the light show of angels and to listen for wind. You told me to watch for fire. You warned me before the swoop and strike of talons. Sometimes, you simply held me, clinging in a long hug like a sleepy koala. And one winter night I awoke with your words in my ears, crystalline: *Don't rule me out.*

As you spoke, your father tossed and sweated beside me. Dan, my beloved. His cold skin drenched our bedsheets. "I'm trying to save our children," came his hoarse voice in the darkness. "They keep falling into their ancestors' graves."

What did you mean, "don't rule me out"? The phrase means to remove from consideration, to prevent. But when you said it, I heard, *Don't take this lightly. Don't make it easier than it is. Don't take one look at me and say, "Forget it." Or "So what?" Take many long looks at me, and at the lives that refract into mine, and decide painstakingly. Decide with all of the care and love and mercy you can find.*

And so, you sent me on this journey.

part one

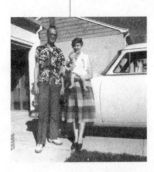

Earl, Esta, and Paula in Pueblo,
Colorado, 1954

That Christmas Eve, I heard my mother go to Luke's bedside. We all knew how deeply my brother slumbered, but I imagined that some part of him must have heard her as she cried softly, "I'm sorry. I'm so sorry."

The dinner dishes were done. The relatives gone. The wineglasses empty. We children, grown, were snug in our beds. Dan and I had just turned out the light in the guest room. In the darkness, sounds were clear. My mother's crying on the other side of the wall reminded me of a night eighteen years earlier, when she had been pregnant with Luke. She had been napping in the afternoon's late-autumn darkness, in the same Seattle house where we now slept. I sat at the kitchen table with my little sister, Amanda. Our father was fixing macaroni. We heard our mother scream.

Scrambling to her bedside, we found her sobbing "Sorry, I'm so sorry" to the bump of her belly. "I shouldn't have been afraid," she wailed as our father switched on the lamps. She said she had seen a yellow angel, three-dimensional like a laser projection, appearing at her side. The angel had seemed purposeful and peaceful as he passed both hands into my mother's belly, straight through walls of skin and muscle and womb. My mother showed us how the angel had rotated his wrists busily inside, fluttering his fingertips like a chef sprinkling something fine.

"I didn't realize what he was doing. When I screamed, the angel turned blue and looked at me, just horrified. It was like he didn't know I was there. He stopped working and just disappeared. I scared him away."

"Right then, I knew," my mother told me years later, "that my baby would have what my dad had." And right then, I knew how she came to believe it was her fault.

When Luke was born, my parents asked the doctor to take a dental X-ray, just to rule out any problems. Later, the pediatrician poked his head into my parents' hospital room and said simply, "There are few tooth buds." My mother and father knew what this meant. A friend had brought a bottle of Champagne, and my father opened it. A nurse then wheeled into the room their pink-faced son with a head of dandelion fluff. My parents looked with love at my brother, who was very quiet and moved his lips with the concentration of an old man, then poured the Champagne. Toasting, they said together, "God's will be done." And they cried long into the night.

Eighteen years later, in 2004, my mother's tears still fell. The guilt of my foremothers haunted me. I had never understood my great-grandmother Josephine's guilt about my grandfather Earl—her eighth child, her baby boy, the chick she kept pulling sadly under her wing. What choice did she have, nearly a century ago? Though she had a brother with the disorder, how could she have known that those traits could appear in her children? Even if she had understood that the disorder was hereditary, could she have prevented a pregnancy if she hadn't wanted to run the risk? Could she have ended a pregnancy she sensed was going wrong? There they were, out on the parched Nebraska farm. The older children would soon leave, and only sisters would remain. Growing older and getting tired, my great-grandparents needed more sons. The snow blanketed and the dust rose and fell and the sunflowers opened and closed. My grandfather Earl, Josephine's too-hot son, was her eighth child and last effort. No one blamed her for Earl's condition, except perhaps her husband, whose back was breaking under all the work his son couldn't do. Little Earl knew, before he knew many things at all, that his mother felt guilty of something. I tried to imagine him going off to kindergarten, already old enough to know that his wisp of a body daily broke his mother's heart.

Earl knew, by the time it mattered, that his medical condition was hereditary, even though he wouldn't know its name until the last decade of his life. A chemist and a medical man, he felt responsible for the biological inheritance of his children. Still, he didn't realize that the gene mutation passed through daughters and appeared in sons. As a father, he must have felt anointed: a healthy, baby-doll daughter and two sweaty, yelping boys. He never knew that the mutation had indeed slipped into the next generation. And he never knew, appraising his robust brood, that they would inherit something else: a sense of abandonment. A lifetime of searching for a trustworthy father, an available mother, solid ground.

By the time my mother married, she suspected she was a carrier of HED. Signs on her body told her there was a risk. She could have adopted children, but that never crossed her mind. And not having children? Hardly an option. To have babies would be my mother's deliverance, or so she hoped. To recover herself from her father's instability, her mother's remoteness, her too-short childhood, she would need to make a family of her own. She would need to till the soil and plant the seeds and nurture and admire the soft-skinned fruits she grew. She would need to love and love and love us, as if to prove it could be done.

My mother's guilt toward Luke, like Josephine's toward Earl, had always seemed unwarranted. Both women, for their own reasons, needed children in order to survive. Beyond abstinence, neither had choices. No gene had been identified. No test had been devised. Not until a decade after Luke's birth would scientists announce that they had discovered the location, on the galactic genomic map, of the HED mutation. Thrilled to tears, my mother called my college dorm room with the news: Women could find out whether they were carriers. Mothers could discover whether their fetuses, or even test-tube embryos, would suffer from the disorder.

But on the day she called with this good news, there was something that neither my mother nor I fully understood. Now, each carrier faced a quandary. Even doing nothing was now deliberate. In preparation for her ethical test, such a woman might learn the stories of her forebears, assigning the events of those lives perhaps undue weight, and then using them as a prism through which to imagine the many possible lives of her many possible children. Eventually, she would need to speak her most private feelings about life and body and motherhood. And later, whether to a doctor or a mother or a brother or a partner or her own child, she would have to answer for her choices.

What would my mother have done if she could have tested her pregnancies? In their marriage, she followed my father into Catholicism. The church's clear morality seemed to suit her, so she might have listened to the pope's edict on abortion and said, "that's that." Or she might have given one moment's thought to the possibility of giving birth to a man like her father, and in a child's terror, emptied her womb. It is a hard question that she cannot answer. It is not, of course, a question of whether she is happy Luke is in the world—that answer is obvious. The question is never about what is. It is about what might have been, and what might be: two things impossible to know.

In 1875 Charles Darwin described a Hindu family affected by a strange disorder: "Ten men, in the course of four generations, were furnished, in both jaws taken together, with only four small and weak incisor teeth and with eight posterior molars. The men thus affected have very little hair on the body and become bald early in life. They also suffer much during hot weather from excessive dryness of the skin." Ectodermal dysplasia, as it was later called, is a single name for a group of about 150 heritable syndromes affecting up to seven in every ten thousand babies born—babies of every ethnicity, mainly boys. Each syndrome has its own signature combination of symptoms. The type of ectodermal dysplasia in my family, X-linked hypohidrotic ectodermal dysplasia, is one of the most common and affects the parts of the ectoderm—an embryonic layer—that shape skin, hair, teeth, fingernails, sweat glands, and parts of the respiratory tree. Boys born with HED exhibit telltale traits: Teeth are few and misshapen. The skin is smooth, firm, dry, nearly hairless. The hair on the head is sparse and often an eye-popping blond. Other hair grows as it should—my brother proved it, growing a strawberry-blond goatee his sophomore year in college.

My grandfather Earl was born with half a dozen tooth buds. My brother had six as well: two on the top and four on the bottom, all conical. A specialist filed and reshaped my brother's natural teeth, fitting him with his first set of dentures at the age of three. Someday, he could choose a painful, transforming surgery to give him dental implants—a full set of teeth embedded in his own gums.

Female carriers of HED also can exhibit some signs of the condition. My mother was missing three adult tooth buds, two on top and one on the bottom. Two unusual conical teeth appeared in her lower jaw when she was about seven years old. I was born with the normal number of teeth. Many of my teeth were small, but not abnormally so. Some grew askance, and my canines came in thick and sharp. One burst through the wall of my upper gums. My dentition was also slow; I was still losing milk teeth in high school. Once all my adult teeth were in place, a year in braces plus cosmetic bonding and a surgery to trim back my gums gave me a sparkling smile that garnered compliments. I felt protective of my newly perfect teeth. Even in high school, I flossed every day.

Neither my grandfather nor my brother was born with the ability to sweat—although sometimes, we learned when he was young, there seemed to be a hint of humidity under Luke's arms. Watching my mother wonder at this, delighting in a wishful possibility, I caught on: We hoped it could still, somehow, not be true.

Nor were my grandfather's or brother's eyes formed with working tear ducts—or, therefore, the ability to cry in the way we all recognize. My mother took great care to explain all of these things to my sister and me, ages three and seven, when she brought Luke home from the hospital. We would be his guardians in the world, when she and my father could not be. As Luke's first summer came on, she carefully schooled us: *Keep him out of the sun. Don't let a babysitter bundle him in blankets. Watch for red ears. Lay him in front of the fan. Give him a soft spray of water—it's better to squirt it onto his skin than into his mouth. When he cries, think heat. Feel his forehead. Tickle him softly in a cool back room.*

Because the ectoderm shapes respiratory tissues, some sufferers of HED have trouble breathing. The linings of the nose and larynx are supposed to be populated with little hairlike cilia, waving in unison to pass sheets of mucus toward the throat. That mucus catches germs and escorts them to the stomach, where they can be harmlessly digested. But HED can cause sufferers to develop comparatively few of those waving cilia and mucus too hard and dry to do its job. My grandfather fought congestion and recurrent pneumonia all of his life, beating infections again and again during childhood. He is said to have spoken very softly. Perhaps this was his elegant refusal of the hoarse voice that many sufferers develop over decades of sinus, throat, and lung infections.

It is possible, I learned as I researched the disorder, that the mutation responsible for HED in our family is associated with another gene problem, about which less is known. This additional defect leads to immunosuppression, adding to a sufferer's onslaught of illness. Perhaps it was this additional defect that caused my grandfather a lifetime of infections, inside and out. Perhaps this extra layer of pain was the demon he fought by self-medicating for decades with a battery of ill-gotten drugs: a last, added battle that likely cost my grandfather his life. There was a chance that it could do the same to my children.

A few months before that Christmas, I had finally summoned the guts to ask my brother to give a sample of his blood. He was just a few weeks into his freshman year of college. My first genetics appointment at the University of Iowa had been a month earlier, and the doctors were waiting to hear whether Luke would participate in the testing process, helping me to find out whether I was a carrier.

I could barely bring myself to dial his number. Luke was supposed to be concerned with college things: playing poker, eating in front of the TV, getting up in time for class. Our communication had waned, so we hadn't been talking much—least of all about HED. As Luke grew up, it had been easy to talk about the disorder because it was simply a practical concern. Babysitting on a hot day, I would ask my brother if he wanted me to dunk his T-shirt in cold water. I would remind him to grab a spray bottle before taking off on a bike ride. When it was time for pajamas, I'd help him slather thick lotion over patches of eczema so he wouldn't scratch and bleed at night. And if he fell asleep in the middle of a late-night showing of *Zorro*, I'd jab him in the ribs until he woke up just enough to spit his dentures into a jar by the sink; he'd get sores if he wore them all night. But eventually, those things became more private affairs. Perhaps around the time my brother first wondered whether a girl would enjoy kissing a guy with false teeth, we stopped talking about his condition. By the time Luke went to college, we were in different worlds. Eight years older than he, I was a graduate student and a year into marriage. I lived in Iowa City; he lived in Seattle. It seemed we had little to talk about.

My call caught him on a weekday afternoon. When he picked up the phone, I felt shame; I had hoped to go through my family planning without Luke ever knowing that Dan and I considered avoiding HED.

"Hi, Sister," he said brightly.

"Hey, I have a really huge favor to ask you," I said.

"Shoot."

"Dan and I have been thinking ahead a little about trying to have a baby sometime in the next couple of years. And now that they know how to find the HED in our blood, Dan and I were thinking that it might be good to find out whether I'm a carrier, so maybe we can try to do some things so our baby won't have it. If we decide that's the right thing to do."

"You can do that?"

"Yeah!" I said, overeager to offer my brother information in trade for a few strands of his DNA. "It would make it a lot easier for them to find out whether I'm a carrier if you could give a sample of your blood first. They'd be able to compare our genes and check to see if mine look like yours."

"That's the favor?"

"Luke, this is really hard for me to ask. I don't want you to think that Dan and I feel like there's something wrong with you. We would be so proud to have a son like you."

He let out a little burst of air. "Bonnie, please. I wouldn't want your kids to have this."

Tension drained out of me. This was, after all, the same kid I stick fought in the backyard all those summers. The same smart, scrappy guy I rassled endlessly while the TV jabbered in the background. The same tender, practical soul who began, as a young boy, protecting his family by concealing the barbs he endured at school. If it could be helped, he never wanted his pain to become anyone else's.

"Let me get this straight," he said. "If your kids didn't get the gene, does that mean none of their kids would have it either? Like you could completely stop it, for all of your kids and grand-kids?"

"Of course."

"Do you know what will happen when I have kids? Could they get the gene?"

"Try not to have any daughters."

Human beings are born with forty-six chromosomes, or bundles of genetic information that tell our bodies, down to the minut-est detail, how to take shape. Half of a person's chromosomes—twenty-three—come from their mother, and the other half from their father.

Of forty-six total chromosomes, every baby receives a single sex chromosome from each parent. Mothers have only Xs to give. Fathers can give either an X or a Y, which determines a baby's sex. A baby who gets an X from her father will be XX: a girl. A baby who gets a Y from his father will be XY: a boy.

The mutation for HED resides on the X chromosome. A father with HED can only pass on the gene mutation if he has a daughter, XX. Since he has only one X to give, and that X carries the mutation, any daughter he has will arrive with HED pro-grammed into her genes. She would show few, if any, signs of the disorder because her body would use her other, healthier X to build her ectoderm—the embryonic layer that becomes skin, hair, teeth, and, in so many ways, identity.

This daughter, then, would have a 50 percent chance of deliv-ering her affected X to a son or daughter of her own. Symptoms would always appear in a son who receives the mutated X; there is no other X for his body to use for certain genetic information.

A daughter who receives the gene mutation would be like her mother: The code for the disorder would be unlikely to harm her, instead waiting quietly to be expressed in a son or grandson.

My great-grandmother Josephine carried this mutation and passed the affected X chromosome to my grandfather Earl. Earl passed that X to my mother, Paula. Paula passed that X to my brother, Luke. And she had a 50 percent chance of passing it to me.

The morning after our Seattle Christmas, and five months since I'd first seen geneticists in Iowa, Dr. Virginia Sybert walked into the exam room where my brother sat with Dan and me.

"Hi, Luke," she said, shaking his hand warmly. She had diagnosed my brother when he was six days old.

"And this is?" she asked, looking at me.

"I'm Bonnie," I said. The doctor's eyes flashed with both recognition and surprise.

"You're beautiful," she said. "Not the girl I remember meeting all those years ago."

When Luke was a toddler, our parents brought the three of us kids to Seattle Children's Hospital to take part in a study of HED. We would each be physically examined for traits of the condition. I remember cringing when I saw a technician take a skin biopsy from my brother's upper arm. Meanwhile, my curly top of a little sister sat adorably while Dr. Sybert pushed through her bouncy ringlets, examining her hair patterns and skin. Amanda didn't seem to be a carrier, the doctor said. And for me, the opposite news.

As we reminisced in the exam room, Dr. Sybert remembered seeing dark circles around my ten-year-old eyes as well as small, slightly crooked teeth. She remembered thin, brittle shafts of straight hair. She was right; I had changed. My teeth had been fixed. With a little extra attention, my hair had become wavy and healthy-looking. I had learned to wear good makeup to show off my green irises instead of the brown crescents under my eyes.

Looking in the mirror, I usually felt satisfied. And with my new-found vanity had come the hope that I wasn't a carrier.

After she chatted with Luke, Dr. Sybert, still with a look of puzzlement, asked if she could examine me. "Please," I nodded.

As the two of us stepped into an empty exam room, a nurse called after us, "Wait! How am I supposed to bill this?"

"It's research," the doctor said.

I took off my winter layers, and she leveled a bright light on my skin. As I stood in my underwear, my hands and feet grew clammy. Would she find a new clue to add to the hints she had seen on my body sixteen years before, bolstering the likelihood that I was a carrier? If she discovered nothing of note, could it mean that my worry was needless? I felt the doctor's breath on my arm and leg hairs as she used cool fingertips to feel, in long, careful strokes, the pores along my limbs. She searched for hair-less patches, for a certain mosaic pattern in my sweat glands. She took my hand in hers and used a flashlight to study the ridges in my fingerprints, assessing the relief between tiny lines. Knowing that HED can cause malformed nipples, I asked about mine. "They look normal to me," she said. Tears suddenly stung my eyes. She was so terribly, gently honest. "You should still be tested," she said. "But I can't say your abnormalities are more than flukes anyone could have."

With hope ballooning in my chest, I returned to sit with Dan in the lobby while Luke had his blood drawn. Moments later, my brother staggered out of the nurse's station, losing his knees, clutching his punctured vein. Then he straightened up, shaking his head and laughing along with Dan at the withering guilt on my face. "I'm not going to die," he said. "Now take me out for breakfast."

My brother's good nature buoyed me, just as it always had. But I couldn't help feeling the heft of the questions begged by the testing we'd begun. My great-grandparents and grandpar-ents, and then my mother and father, had all made their babies on faith. They knew HED ran in their bloodline, at least as far back as Josephine's mother, and there was nothing to do about it but pray. But now, not even two decades after Luke's birth, perhaps "God's will" was no longer a force Dan and I had to accept. "What is *our* will?" we had been asking, trying to be ready for anything.

Even if I turned out to be a carrier, it would be possible for us to ensure a healthy biological child. We could pay tens of thousands of dollars for in vitro fertilization, followed by preimplantation genetic diagnosis to identify unaffected embryos. Or we could begin a pregnancy in the privacy of our bedroom. Near the end of the first trimester, I could undergo chorionic villus sampling, or CVS, to have our fetus tested for the HED mutation—and possibly face an excruciating choice.

As Dan and I drove with Luke back to my parents' house to gobble holiday cookies, my unease continued. The more I thought about the blood test, the more disturbed I felt. I knew I was entering uncharted waters. If I turned out to be a carrier, it would mark a new age in my family's genetic pedigree. Mine would become the generation of the test, the choice. Women hear all the time that they must look back to discover their family's destructive cycle and then break it. I saw a pattern of guilt in the carrier mothers before me. How could I shed the guilt of passing an affected X chromosome to my child, when I would be the only one of these women with a true choice? My mother and my great-grandmother had the option of releasing their guilt by accepting that sons with HED were fated for them: God's will. But with the answers available to our generation, Dan and I knew that having a son with HED would mean we chose it for him.

paula

You were only one when your grandfather died. I had nightmares about him all the time. He would fall on me, and I would be afraid his needles would jab me. Even though he was dead, it seemed like he could still wreck my life whenever he wanted to. I was a new mother, and I had this sense of power, but every time I saw his face, I felt afraid and furious and sad, just like when I was little. I was still looking for a real father, and I still wished that somehow we could go back to the days in Broomfield, Colorado, where the only bad thing I remembered was the time Greg stomped a crawdad, and its blood came out yellow like mustard. Or even Greeley, an hour north of Broomfield, where Greg held my hand as we skated on the neighborhood pond, and I looked up into the snowflakes, believing I could become one. All the time I was growing up, I felt like it was possible for our family to find that sweet innocence and simple life again. If my mom could just build my dad up enough for him to quit doing drugs. If my dad could just catch some better luck. But I was always disappointed. And even after he was gone, he kept making messes of my days.

Sometime after I had you two girls, I finally had a happy dream about my dad. It was a sunny, windy day. He was driving down a highway toward a beautiful bridge, this huge span over the water. He came to a tollbooth, and I saw him pay, and then he just smiled and waved and drove off without looking back. As though he finally knew what he was supposed to be doing. I didn't dream about him for a long time after that. But then after Luke was born, I was sitting on the bed in my room, nursing him. I must have been falling asleep, and a vision came out of nowhere: I saw my dad peek through the window. I screamed. His expression was so offended, as if he only wanted to see his grandson. But I jumped up and shooed him away: "Get out of here! Don't you dare look at us!"

Your dad and I have both been dreaming about him. Maybe he keeps coming back because all these years we've been telling the story wrong, and it rattles his bones. He wants to tell his version now. You are part artist and part scientist. Maybe you were meant to show us what happened.

As the tail of winter blustered around our Iowa bungalow, my brother's DNA crawled through tests. My subconscious filled with ghosts. My dreams were becoming like my mother's: vivid, complex, somehow creeping into the waking hours. A picture of my young grandfather—optimistic, tortured, ephemeral—had begun to form in my mind. In my peripheral vision, shapes of his body flickered across landscapes of the past. I saw my grandmother Esta, too: a vibrant young nurse. And my mother, a sprite in an Easter dress. In my dreams, I unpacked boxes of yellowed artifacts, discovering old photos that no one in my family had ever seen. With my eyes closed, I gazed out over prairie wheat, feeling mixed among generations. Some nights, I felt the pull of Earl's ghost so strongly that it frightened me. He seemed to be above me, in the batty attic, and below me, in the chilly basement. I didn't know what to say to him, or how to explain my growing obsession with his life, or how to justify the fact that my digging seemed to have disturbed his spirit. I was the only grandchild he ever knew. Would he appreciate the light I was shining into his grave, or would he tell me I had no business trying to decipher the faded script of his life? Earl had always been a pariah. If he never could make himself understood to the people closest to him, what business did I have assuming I could do better? One night, as I drifted to sleep, I saw the smooth arch of his high forehead, his saddle nose, and his lips, which were brown for a white man's lips and pillowy small. *Speak to me,* I begged. But he didn't say a word. He simply stared beyond me.

I wanted more. I needed to examine his life. To see it through his own stinging eyes, from within his fevered skin.

earl

My first grandchild. Your mother lays you in my arms, and I look into your face. You open your eyes. You open your mouth. I think you might cry. But you don't make a sound.

"Shh," I, whisper "sh, shh: a secret for you. Here's the special thing I brought. I had a lady in my building make it. I picked out the pink for you, and even the pattern for the quilting. If your mama uses it and wraps it around you all the time, you'll think nothing ever felt so soft and fresh. It's silk. Silk is always cool. See, cool to your chin, just like that."

That's love. Mother's hand, always so cool on my neck. "Sh, shh, Earl," my mother would say, "you hush now. It's only a gull. You're a big boy now. Eight years old."

But the gulls, all of them trailed me, and I felt like a little whitefish beneath them. They swooped and dove at the worms churned into sunlight behind the plow, and the dust powdered their feathers brown, and they blinked and dropped like newspapers, and I felt them falling at me. The time I saw a dead one, I thought it was my brother's shirt. I stopped the tractor, and I walked over and reached down, and it was dirty. Eyes blue-white and covered with flies.

"Sh, shh," my mother said. Her hands so cool.

I stayed away from the chickens, too, but after all, they were only chickens and common. The gulls I hated, though, and the pigeons and crows. My sisters knew if they found dead feathers they could fling them in my face and get me good.

Sisters. In the kitchen they said, where it was hot, hot with canning tomatoes, "Mother, we'd like to go to the lake beach now if that's all right."

Mother with a scarf on her head and dripping by the steam.

"Sure you can," she said. "And take your brother."

"But Mother, he's so ugly, do we have to?"

They told truth. My eyes were so light, I squinted as the sun seared red the lids and the tops of my cheeks. My ribs sprung out, but my stomach caved in. My hair was so thin, it blew without wind. My big brother's britches hung on me with a length of rope, and my skin was so dry, it itched and sizzled up in hard pink patches. I could have said to my sisters, "Least I don't smell, since I don't sweat."

But I opted not to open my mouth, for my teeth were only six and pointed. While my brothers and sisters sang, I leaned in the doorway, hiding naked gums behind my lips. I didn't mind waiting out the twilight there, while my mother jabbered the piano keys and they all howled and laughed. I could smile downright delightful with my mouth closed. And it was delight I felt.

Then, when I was an older boy, I could choose. At the garden end of the near section, my father grew a patch of popping corn. He popped it for us under a crop-fire moon. It was up to me: wear my new dentures and leave the hard popcorn or float the fragile teeth in a glass of water, where they watched me like a weird watery promise, and try to crack away at the buttery kernels with everyone else. I kept my teeth in my mouth, though I wanted to eat with the whole family so merry. The more I wore them, the more clearly I learned to speak, my tongue mapping its way along new shelves and ridges and walls. The more I wore them, the less they drifted and glinted and clicked.

"Smile," my mother told me, two papery hands holding my face. "*Smile* me that beautiful smile."

After school when the sun screamed, I shot hoops on the barn, perfecting. I kept a shirt floating in a bucket of water, and I swapped when the one I wore burned dry. Sometimes at sunset the wind changed and puffed light and cold, and I could shoot hoops with a dry shirt on as long as I wanted, the stars finding their needle holes and the cows shifting on their feet and breathing on their babies, home for sleep.

"You're no invalid," my mother always said, a lyric to grow by.

But when I came to his side in the barley, my father said, "You go inside now. Just go inside with your mother." He turned away, and drops tumbled from his dark hair, sopped together like paintbrush tips. I saw my brothers, their muscles rippling brown and shining. In the ice barn I cooled down. Sitting on a frozen block, I watched through a crack in the door: the wheat waving and the sky pale and tall. The windmill croaking and my mother there at the pump. The gurgle of water, black in the earth. My father pushed open the door and said, "Look, son, really. You're meltin' a pants seat there. Go with your mother in the house."

In the house in the cellar. Preserves jars red and blue, applesauce and peaches. Pickles and tomatoes and cold hard dirt to relax the soles of my feet. There was nothing to look at, but it didn't matter when I went down there so blazing white-eyed from the sun that I couldn't see and I was just lucky not to squash my toes on the dead deer mice.

On that farm I saw my mother slick with sweat and butchering a pig, glancing at me with a deep, sad pain. I saw my brothers worry over coins and hope for farms of their own. I saw my sister in love with a woman—the fast flush of her cheeks, the parting of her lips—though she thought no one knew. I didn't mind living in a town where everyone knew Earl was sickly—awful sickly—and born that way, ain't it a shame. I didn't mind playing until I nearly died when the basketball team needed me. I was taller than most of the guys, and I could think while I moved. The thing I did mind: in the middle of my joke, just when a girl was ready to smile, feeling sudden lava in my neck and needing to stop my voice, slink away, slump down, find a shadow, drench my head, wait to see if I would live or die. And whether she would stay for the punch line.

When my oldest brother graduated high school, Dad said to him, "Come on, Son. We'll go downtown and have dinner; you'll join the Elks tonight."

When my next brother graduated, Dad said, "Welcome, Son, to the Order of Elks."

There I was, salutatorian of my graduating class, and my father said to me, "So long, Son. Write your mother."

It was better that I left. At the Colorado State College of Education and at Greeley General Hospital, no one squinted in search of my eyelashes. No one gaped when I yawned and my dentures showed. They were more worldly; many in my circle were medical people. There in Greeley, before they knew me as a sickly boy, they knew me as a chemist. Before I was weak, I was heroic—an ambulance driver. Before I was slow to chew and swallow, I was quick to make them laugh. Before I was needy, I was an orderly giving help and comfort. Before they considered my problems breathing, they saw my problems steering: a happy parade of dents along the bumper of my Pontiac. I became nice and fat under my chin, and my stomach certainly didn't protrude, but it no longer caved in. I manned the bar at hospital parties, and young doctors raised their glasses to me. And the girls watched me. Jack took a photo I love, where I'm handing Dr. Wheeler a cup—Dr. Wheeler with his thick black hair and his big green eyes and handsome square ears like my brothers'. Wheeler is smiling at me and so are all four girls. The girls are watching me, and my mouth is open, telling them the thing that is making their faces crush with laughter.

In the halls of Greeley General, I wore white. I moved bed-pans, and I moved people. I laid sacks of sand against the feet of polio patients, who needed their muscles to find certain angles in order to keep their strength. I shaped the sand so their calves could stretch. But sand, always shifting. Weeks would pass, and I'd see those feet drop to the sides and stiffen, the legs go twisted and hard.

Esta, a nurse in her own bright white. She brushed my arm in the cafeteria. She smoked on the lawn with the other girls, and I watched the cigarettes touch her fingers, her fingers touch her mouth. Esta, too, shook her head to see the polio patients withering. She might be moved, I thought. So I drew, I built, I wrote my application. My design, the Adjustable Foot Rest for Polio Bed Patients, received U.S. Patent 2,720,878. "It's not a complicated thing," I shrugged when she tried not to look too impressed. "Somebody just had to sit and make it."

And next, for the dry, dry air in hospital rooms where patients with tired passages coughed and bled, the Aerosol Humidifier Apparatus, U.S. Patent 2,696,210.

Doctors were using old-style nebulizers with big glass bulbs, designed to press medicine into lungs. The bulbs would become bacterial with use and reuse. And they were thin walled. I watched a doctor's hand slip, shattering glass all over a patient's face as she gasped for air. At home, I worked up a design for the plastic Nebulizer. When I showed it to Dr. Helman, anesthetist, he nodded and said, "That's something you've got there, son."

As an orderly, it was not uncommon for me to roll cadavers. In the elevators, if we were alone, sometimes I looked. I pushed down the sheets and looked at their faces. Sometimes blue and anguished, more often pale and long, empty like dusty wine glasses. Quite often the eyes were open, wheeled back. Sometimes a smell of paste reached me, antiseptic and starchy, a glue unloosed. The thing I noticed most when I pushed them to the elevators, looking past the peaks of their tented noses and pressing the down button to the morgue, was their shocking weight. Even on wheels, death is a staggering heft. Except when I rolled a baby. When I rolled a baby, it wasn't the weight of death that slowed me, but the mother's wails. They hooked my ears, holding me back.

I worked at the funeral home and attended the night phones and drove the ambulance. I lived in the apartment below the parlor where they laid out the dead. When Junior and Calhoun came over to drink beer and choke the night with laughter, I don't think we ever forgot those heavy heads on their satin pillows upstairs. At night I dreamed that bodies crashed through the floor, and those limbs like stone trapped my limbs, and no scream would come from my dry little throat.

Sometimes there was a scream barely caught in Junior, too—I could see it in his eyes. Once on campus I asked him, before I knew: "How's your folks?"

"Got no folks," he said right there, with the green grass brimming and the daffodils open. "Was two years old sittin' at the table drinking my milk. Mother was fixing breakfast. Saw her bend down into the stove and the fire caught up her gray sleeve, and I watched the fire climb her like spines up a dragon tail, and soon my mother was a blaze whirlin'. My brothers and my sister pulled me outta the house, and the whole house, we watched it burn and burn from the street till it was black and there was nothin' left, not even my mother. My dad sent me to my aunt, and then he died of cancer, and my aunt passed me down to my brother Art who raised me the rest the way up. Never forget my mother whirlin' fire like that and screamin'."

In the park one of our young nights, I went to the keg and filled my beautiful stein with black enamel night and curling lime vines and drowsing peach blossoms. A ketchuppy corn dog hung between my teeth as the beer foamed cold down the side of my mug and fell puttering by my shoes. Esta came up. I smelled her by my side, a sparrow's nest and peppermint. She said, "Earl Hickman . . . whaddaya know?" That little tone of hers. She already knew anything I could have told her. Little, bright gray eyes and red, red lips. She wrapped her fingers around my stein, and I followed her into the trees.

When she told me the news a month later, she watched my eyes to see if I was ready. I saw her thinking, *Too young. He's a baby, just twenty-three.* But I smiled and held my words simple and plain and honest: "Oh, that's such wonderful news."

She waited, so I said also, "I'm so happy."

I did feel a tremor. But I loved Esta so much. I asked her, "How do you feel?"

"Happy," she said. "I love little babies."

It was your mother inside her. Going to be a baby just like you.

"When will it come?" I asked her.

"March," she said.

It was July and smoldering: wheat harvest time, when all of us went back to the farm to work. So Esta and I decided to get married there, in Bushnell, Nebraska. Then for our honeymoon, we'd drive to her parents' farm in Alberta, where I could meet the old Estonians and they could hear the baby news.

There was hubbub in my parents' house. My mother looked tall that day and waited in the living room. Jack was there, the friend who always watched me closely. He watched my heart right through my eyes and loved me. We stood by the back bedroom door where Esta dressed. I said to Jack, "You know, here I am at my wedding, and we all know what comes after marriage. But if you were brought up with these medical conditions I have, you'd think a dozen times about having kids of your own. We know it's hereditary. It gives you pause."

Then we heard Esta's girlfriends. Swannie said, "Listen, you don't have to marry him, you know."

"I love this guy!" Esta hissed in her citrus way.

Lois said, "Then tell us. Tell us."

So she told them. "Well, he's tall and he loves sports and he invents and he's careful and we have such a good time together. We laugh."

"More," said Swannie.

Esta sighed and sounded bored. "We sat by Glenmere Lake in the park on the orange blanket, and he said, 'I like orange, don't know why.' I said, 'Me too.' He took his shirt off and I had a swimsuit on so my own back was bare. First I touched his skin and felt it softly, and I popped the pimples on his back when I found them. And then he did mine. Finally I said, 'Okay, enough, quit pawing around back there.' That reminded him of a little song: *Well where oh where is dear little Esta? Where oh where is dear little Esta? Way down yonder in the paw paw patch. Away down yonder in the paw paw patch . . .* And he sang it right at me with goofy bug eyes, and he just made me laugh and laugh. Then we just tipped back on the blanket and breathed and breathed. He whispered, *Picka paw paw, put it in yer pocket,* and I started another fit until I was too tired to even smile anymore. There were big brown and yellow houses all around us, and I said, 'Wouldn't it be something to have one of these houses?' And he said, 'You bet.'"

So Lois said to her, "All right, Esta. But you know you don't have to. We can take care of each other."

"How do you feel?" Swannie asked.

And Esta told them, "You ninnies. I feel rich like the bottom of the ocean."

I heard my sisters let up a cackle in the living room. Everyone sounded happy. And soon there was Esta, almost my wife. Her brown hair and white dress. We stood by the cake and said our vows. She didn't look at me. Probably because of the secret we had. Maybe she thought we would burst out laughing. Everyone clapped, and we kissed. I watched her looking into the cake, concentrating so hard on the frosting, the loops and swirls. I couldn't eat it and neither could she—maybe that was why I couldn't. She held the heavy silver server in her hand, staring down, and I saw her wan face reflected.

Sitting at her parents' table in Barons, it was wheat out the windows, like the views I had known all my life. But in Alberta the horizon looked farther away, or maybe just looking north it seemed the earth curved harder. On the drive up, Esta taught me to say, *hello, how are you?* and *thank you* in Estonian. We sat there in the kitchen. Her mother had a pastry full of cheese and sugar on the table. It steamed like the day. I kept waiting because they didn't reach for it yet, not one of them.

I knew Esta was doing a fine job of telling them about us. I couldn't understand a word. I sat up straight—my posture being something to admire. I knew she was saying to them, in their old song of a language, *He's an inventor and a genius, and he'll be making plenty of money in the new job for us, because a precious baby is coming. The new job is with Winthrop Laboratories, selling drugs to doctors, and he can send you medications, too, if you need them. Samples, you know. And he's got a beautiful car, hasn't he? And he knows wheat farms because he grew up this way, too.*

The sun beat hard there, but the breeze was cooler than home. I moved grain bins with her father, Hans, while Esta and Julene gathered eggs and milked the *lehma*—I think she said *lehma* meant "cows." Hans was shaped like a block, and his mouth was set; the creases ran deep. I didn't know what his grunts meant, or his lips moving soundless while his eyes scanned the granary. But I liked him. I liked Esta's proud and jaw-certain parents. They worked like people who had three pretty daughters and never knew the blessing of even one strong son and never for a moment cared.

Esta brought me into the henhouse. It tasted like chicken droppings, thick in the little hot square of air. But Esta said it also tasted like girlhood and grain, like scattering feed when new sun glittered on the wet wheat. She said it tasted like sisters and jumpers and a bonnet tied under the chin. Three girls ran around that farm in their frocks, growing brown like horses and hens. It was Esta's job to gather the eggs, counting. Inside she would ask her mother, "How many this time?" And her mother might guess, "*Kaheksakümmend? Kaheksakümmend üks?*" And if her guess was off, Esta got to keep the extra eggs and sell them for pocket change. Her mother put each day's egg money in a pot. If she could get up the courage, she went to the bank in the village where they didn't understand Estonian, and she would deposit the egg money into an account. When Julene was too bashful to take her money to the bank, she would send a daughter instead. It had to be done; a generation of egg money saved would provide a comfortable old age.

I followed Esta inside, the eggs in her apron. She asked, "How many, Mum?" and Julene laughed low and charmed, because in a flash she saw my wife without lipstick: a girl in a berry-stained smock, not a grown woman in a tight-waisted dress, growing her grandbaby.

I took your grandmother to Pueblo, Colorado, and started my new job with the drug company. I drove all over three states. The road was long, gray in winter. In Wyoming the grasses were dead and the trees were naked, and day after day I carried my case and went to see the doctors in their little wood-paneled offices. I had a bad cold that Christmas, 1953, and Esta said, "Take the cough syrup." It had been a long time since I'd needed cough syrup. It perked me up—I couldn't believe how. So I started keeping a bottle in the car, on the seat beside me. I bought more every few days when I ran out. Because when I arrived at those doctors' offices on those bleak Mondays and Tuesdays and Wednesdays, still so far from home and comfort, I didn't want to be gravelly-sounding. Or shy. I needed to be chipper and upbeat and confident and, yes, full of courage and knowledge and charisma because they had to have faith in me. They had to remember me as delightful and eager and like a breath of fresh air. They had to think, "This young man sure is pert. What an ace," or I would fail my family.

And Esta deserved me fresh and bright, too. If it had been spring, she could have planted peas. If it had been summer, she could have hosed our brand-new lawn. But it was winter and gloomy, and she was now far from the hospital and the other nurses, her girlfriends. I went four weeks on the road, came a couple weeks back, then went another four or five weeks away. On my returns I would come through the door with rain, or snow, on my hat and sing out, "My bird!"

Once she stood by the stove in tears. Alone so often, she had forgotten how much rice and fish to buy for two. She looked at the meal she had made, and looked at me as if remembering my size, and looked down at her round belly, and knew she had made too little.

I was a hundred miles away when things started. It was only January. She should have been writing her sister or chopping carrots or shopping for baby blankets, but instead she answered the phone breathing breathing breathing. Weeks and weeks too soon. I drove and prayed. They let me see my wife, just to tell her I was there. It was just before the girl came out, and I saw a flash in Esta's eyes: *Dog. You did this, you dog.* Despite her tiny size, the baby's coming still frightened my wife and made her howl and moan.

I stood in the waiting room. Would someone come down the hall, before I could even see her, and cover her face? Cover my daughter's face? I had seen them do it. Orderlies, nurses. I had seen them come in and realize it even before the family, and they cover the dead baby's face. My miniature girl.

Our lace-fingered daughter weighed four pounds the day she was born. Esta told me that she had named her Paula and chose Julene for a middle name after her mother. I filled out the birth certificate on the first day, and there was my last name attached to a new human. She weighed three pounds the day after she was born and two pounds the following morning. Esta packed her suitcase to go home. The nurse said to me, "Sir, you might like to hold your daughter. At least this once. In case." So I walked next to the tray and there she was, looking sunbaked somehow. The nurse lifted her, sliding her fingertips under each end, and laid her in the palm of my right hand. I put my left hand alongside, to catch a little arm reaching. That little arm was smaller than my thumb. Just as long, but thinner.

Your mother was a tiny baby doll. Her eyes were just lines, meeting somewhere above her nose. When she opened her mouth it was littler than a penny. She sounded like a newborn tiger, alien and strong. The nurse thought it might be the last time. But two pounds felt heavier than I had imagined, and when I felt the mass of her, and her sticky sweat, I knew she was real and staying. Two days later, we brought her home.

Esta had her company then—a wailing girl who never slept. I heard Esta talking to our baby doll as I drove those bleak roads. *You are the littlest thing! Just the littlest thing! You scared your mama and your papa, but you knew, didn't you? You knew. Where is your papa? Where is that man? On the road, on the road, singing down the road. He is singing down the road for you, his baby, baby doll. What's he singing? What's he singing? He is singing diapers and bottles and bottles and diapers and crying and crying and rocking her rocking her, his little baby doll. But does your papa know a diaper? Does your papa hold the bottle? Of course not, because he is singing down the road with a trunk full of medicine, and he's going the other way. When your papa comes home does he give your little skin a bath? Does he push the bottle past your lips? Of course not, no, but what does he do? He rocks you in your little wooden cradle, and you don't cry, you don't cry, you don't cry.*

A ghost lullaby followed me everywhere. Over the rangelands, into the service stations, through the motel key slots, down the clinic corridors. The doctors believed they knew me, winning as I was. But they didn't know I was tired, passing through Kansas, the circles beneath my eyes growing darker each day. They didn't know that I was hardly ever in bed with my wife. That my baby doll was finally getting bigger, and already I couldn't remember the heft of her, three days old in my hand. I sat right in their exam rooms, and they could see me fine. But the doctors didn't notice the pain in my eyes, young and bitter as spring radishes. They could not know the way the bridge of my nose pressed down so hard between my eyes that I could barely breathe in the stuffy, hot car through the dry winter wind. That my nasal spray was gone again, and whenever I bought more it was gone again just as quickly. That even the spray did nothing for me anymore. The air still burned and trampled through.

I came through the door on a sunny afternoon in June, and like always, I called for my bird and my baby doll. The air was in odd pieces though, and things were everywhere. There was no meal. The baby cried in the living room. Esta came from the bathroom, wet lipped. "I have supper for you," she said to me, "but I want broth. Oh you girl," she said, picking up our daughter, "You cry cry cry. We are trying this again, little girl," she said, without looking at me. "A March baby, like you were supposed to be."

I stood there still wearing my hat, too warm, flushed with pleasure and confusion. The house was a scatter, and so were our heads. I just kept standing, a slow smile finding me, then finding Esta, until I could take one step and slide my hand around the low part of her back. I felt her soften, and then I knew I could kiss her, and kiss her, until she looked at our baby, embarrassed.

"I have stuffed cabbage leaves," she said. "It sounds good now. With a tomato. A salty, hot tomato slice on top."

I took a step back from Esta, holding our daughter, and the sun hit the child's hair, and suddenly I saw how blond she was. "My little baby doll," I said, taking her. "Your hair is practically white!"

I sat down and put her on my knee. And my wife saw the baby suddenly and said, "My! How cute she really is!"

Dr. Helman had encouraged my Nebulizer project from the beginning. "You just get that patent through, Earl," he said, "and you let me know, and we can start production. You'll be on your way. We'll make plenty of money. I have no doubt, so I will promise to get things started with a little capital, but most of the proceeds from sales will be yours, of course—you've done all the hard work lining up manufacturers and distributors anyway."

His words were fuel. I worked late every night through the summer, at my desk in the hall, drawing, drafting letters, writing the patent application—one longer and more complex than the others had been. "This is going to be big, Esta," I told her. "I just have to pull it all together and put in for the patent, and then we could be set for life. But I have to finish. You have to let me finish. Don't hover in the doorway like that. Go to sleep and open the windows by the bed and let a little of this blue slow summer in."

It stayed that way for two years. Even after we moved north to Broomfield, proof the money was beginning to come. She always wanted to know what I was doing. I wasn't taking as many road trips, because the Nebulizer was a better investment of my time. She worried. And she was lonely for me. But we had our friends and the neighbors next door. Esta and Joyce sat out with the little ones on the lawn almost every summer day. "Here are the two blond babies in their swimsuits," I would hear my wife say. "You babies stay away from the house, that hot white wall! Yes, come over and play under the hose! Paula, come play in the water. No, Greggy's still too small. You run through. Run through, big girl. You love those pretty roses, don't you? Pink and yellow. Say *pink and yellow*! When will we ever get a peep from you? Listen to that loud Greggy! What a loud boy! He's hungry. Time for a cookie, Paula? No? My, but you're a sweaty girl, aren't you? Aren't you? Just like your brother. Now there's a smile!"

I loved the way she gave this to the breeze, to me, idly listening. Days before, as I went out the door with my suitcase, she clutched my sleeve with a trembling hand. She whispered: "Joyce said Paula should have more teeth by now. All of them! Was there something I did wrong? Were there vitamins I should have taken?"

I knew by her look—of tenderness for me and pleading—that she was asking if Paula had inherited my condition. A shadow did cross my eyes. But no, I could tell her softly, no. "She sweats a little, doesn't she?"

"Yes, oh, plenty!"

"She's all right," I said, heavy, passing out the door for the road again in the white heat.

And now on my return, as they all played on the lawn, our kids and Joyce and Jim's, Esta offered those workaday mother words into the air, a reminder to the breeze and me: *All is well.*

Esta had Joyce then, and all of her letters with her sisters, and I still had my guys, Junior and Calhoun. They were the brothers I wished for. In some ways they were like my brothers back on the farm—they fought in Korea while I stayed home sweatless. But they were also better than my farm brothers because when they came back from overseas they drove straight down to see me. When Calhoun got back from flying in Korea, he married Betsy and had a daughter—she was the same age as Paula. He was good with my kids. Said, "Hello, Yellow!" whenever he saw Paula on the porch with her light hair blowing. Calhoun's cheeks were squared off, set fierce, but his handsome, old black eyes still gave me this look that said, "Earl, you old dodgery dog, you're always such a surprise."

And Junior, he was a first-rate chemist. So in the army they thought it would be a good joke to put him in as a chef in the mess. He played along all right—that was always his way. He came home still smiling odd as ever, with his short trunk thicker than before. Always wearing his white T-shirt and khakis. He never had a girl. When he came over, he'd say ever so softly to my wife, in almost a whisper, "How do you do, Esta." Hard to imagine why this pleased her so much that she'd suddenly be chopping the onions so much slower. But it was harmless, I knew.

Calhoun always made me want to fly and loop through the sky and shoot into a crowd of admirers, all of them chanting, *Thank-you-He-ro, thank-you-He-ro.* Junior made me want to heat a can of soup, light a fire, bring a blanket for his big soft shoulders. Together the three of us just sparred and laughed. Laughed so much. But that didn't mean we couldn't be serious for each other. They had their needs. I had mine. Esta would let us have the living room for hours, even when Paula and Greg were fussing, trying to fall asleep. Sometimes she sat in there and drank with us. Sometimes she turned the pages of her magazines at the kitchen table. Sometimes she had rollers in her hair or painted her nails, and she didn't even care if the fellas saw. As I said, they were like brothers.

And of course there was Helman, who was more like a father. A few years passed, and we had the Nebulizer, U.S. Patent 2,785,923. He was paying me fair from sales, and I could feel his pride in me, his young charge, a budding businessman, a sudden expert in the delivery of pharmaceuticals to the lungs. He sat in my wife's kitchen, still encouraging me: "You should invest it, Earl. I want to give you some ideas. I'm looking for a partnership up in Greeley, a real estate partnership, and I was telling my wife on Sunday, I said, 'You know, I should see about that Earl Hickman, see if he wants a part in this. Maybe he can even run things, be president of the corporation. He's got the brains of an elephant, focused and never forgetting.' Anyway, Earl, you should think of investing your earnings with me. If you do, there'll be heaps more by Christmas. You could get one of those houses up in Greeley, the ones you're always talking about."

I was hungry for all of that. But Esta pulled back. Happy in Broomfield with her friends. Lounging out front in the sun with Joyce, the kids tromping like we didn't know what. In and out of their little pools, past the lawn chairs, sprinting with sliding popsicles and comic books and bucketfuls of crawdads from the park creek. Esta and Joyce would keep their magazines spread on their laps but never read them. They smoked and talked about Khrushchev visiting, and the Luna, and Castro being a few cards short of a deck, and the new missile silo going in just one county north. *Whhh*, my wife would blow out slow, such lovely cars going by in her sunglasses.

We had dreamed of Greeley, but to see her then, she was home. She loved to sit in our kitchen on a simple red chair beneath the turquoise phone, knowing it would ring, a cigarette in her hand as she watched the whole inside of the house—from that one spot, she could see Greg on the living room floor with his chin pointed up at the cartoons and also watch Paula sorting books under the kitchen table. And soon the phone would jangle, and it would be Joyce from next door, saying "Sorry, Esta, I know I ought to just run right over instead of calling, but the boys got into the blueberries and I have a mess here, but I had to say real quick I hope you and Earl are still planning to come over for supper and pinochle. The kids can play outside. It's going to be a warm night I think, the first one of the year."

It was too warm that spring. We ordered concrete poured. Both families were going to have nice new driveways. Building the forms wasn't bad, the crickets just starting to hatch and the mornings cool. But the day the concrete came, I had to wrap a wet towel around my head before I could even start to rake that thick, heavy mix. I pushed and pushed, but my eyes started to twitch, and I couldn't see that I wasn't doing any good. I heard Jim say, "Y'all right, Earl?" But I didn't know any words for how to answer, and instead I just walked inside. I probably left my rake out there, sinking in. Had to see if it would be cool on my bedspread if I lay there with my bare back on it. I closed my eyes. After the sun went down and the mayflies came out, I would go see if the concrete could budge.

"Daddy," Paula said. Without opening my eyes I could see her, a ribbon of child at my bedside. "Daddy, Mom says you're too hot."

"That's right," I whispered. "Too hot."

"But Daddy, Jim's not too hot, and he's still workin'."

"I know, Baby Doll," I told her slow. "It's different for every-body." I needed to turn over, to cool my chest and stomach. I hoped the bedspread still had cold spots. "You go play now," I said. "Stay out of that gray mud."

Yet it was only that night, as I finished smoothing our drive-way, that I believed my condition was sometimes, only some-times, a gift. There I was, outside alone, hearing the sink and kitchen clatters from all the yellow window squares of all the happy houses. In ours, my wife and daughter and son were put-ting clean plates away. In another, Joyce stood, and I watched Jim washing his hands in the kitchen, about to get walloped with a towel for that. And their two boys, wheeling around their par-ents' legs, screeching wild. I smelled our food coming from their house, Joyce fixing spaghetti for all of us. The sky over the field across Main Street was purple, and the other way, behind our houses, was pink streaked with blue, and the dog stood there with me. He saw this every night as he rested on the lawn: quiet street, winkered sky, electric houses, whole little families clumped like magnets. I hosed off the rake, the wind of insect wings brushing my arms.

part two

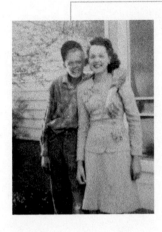

Earl and Sadie on the family farm
in Bushnell, Nebraska, circa 1944

In the summer of 2004, before my first genetics appointment, and before asking my brother for his blood sample, I had been wondering if life could get any better. I had been married for almost a year to my best friend. We were graduate students, and our summer days seemed clipped from a midwestern living magazine. Elm leaves waved over our little brown bungalow, fanning away the July swelter as we stretched our bare feet from the porch swing in the mornings. Chattering sprinklers, droning lawn mowers, and whirring cicadas wove a comforting soundtrack through the humid afternoons. The house wrens had finally quelled their spring prattle, cardinals belled lustily for mates, and barred owls questioned their lovers in the moonlight.

Dan and I loved to sit on our little backyard deck after sundown. We caught fruitsicle drips with our tongues and nudged away mosquitoes as we watched the show: a coliseum of fireflies blinking green, blue, and orange. They rose from the lawn up into the peonies, drifting higher through the redbud and lilac, finally ornamenting the tips of the evergreens along our rambling dirt alleyway. It reminded us of darkened football stands erupting with camera flashes.

Most evenings, I took it in slowly, with half-closed eyelids, sitting very still with my luck: a strong, handsome young husband, a sturdy house framed by flower beds, an orange clown of a cat, and a green garden clambering with tomatoes, zucchini, and corn.

It might have been enough, but like my mother, I couldn't imagine a childless life. I had just made a doctor's appointment for a month later, in August. I would meet with a genetic counselor and a physician, describe my family pedigree, discuss the disorder, and eventually submit to blood tests in order to learn my status. If the news returned that I carried HED, Dan and I would have a battery of decisions before us.

I had been feeling a tug from the West, a beckoning from my grandfather's Nebraska gravesite. I wasn't sure what I would find there, but I sensed there was a story waiting—something that would give me guidance if my test results returned with the marker for HED. Dan and I had been considering a summer trip to the Rockies, and it occurred to me that we should drive instead of fly.

"So," I said, trying not to crack the night's calm, "How about a road trip? We could make some stops in Nebraska and Wyoming and Colorado on our way to the mountains. I'm thinking of retracing my mom's childhood and trying to find out more about her dad."

I turned, squinting to see his twilit expression.

"We could do that," he said.

My husband required little persuasion to undertake an adventure— even someone else's. So, the next day, he requested time off from his summer job. Our next-door neighbor agreed to feed the cat and water the garden. I stopped the mail and the paper. And a few days later, home a little early, Dan scurried down the basement stairs to gather up the tent, sleeping bags, and camp stove. He packed the ice chest and loaded the car. Half amused and half baffled, he watched me fill the trunk with family photo albums, books, files, and phone numbers. Like me, he believed that our journey was important without knowing exactly why.

He took the driver's seat and handed me a map. For our first night, we planned to drive eight hours across most of Iowa and Nebraska, pitching our tent at the leading edge of the near-arid landscape that early explorers called the Great American Desert. The freeway sang beneath our little white Civic as the low sun made the windshield blaze. We munched sandwiches, listened to music, sang, chatted, and then rode in silence, wondering where we were going and what we would find. Midnight approached, and we cranked the music to keep awake. When we finally stopped to sleep on the bank of the Platte River, a ruddy moonlight hugged the flat prairie all around us.

In the morning, it looked like rain. The sky had filled with the mucky plains thunderheads we had learned to recognize in our first year away from our native western Washington. Slinging the tent and sleeping bags into the trunk, we sailed on, in the opposite direction of the storm, passing right beneath it. On the other side, the sky opened into a surprising thin blue. The air lost its humidity as we climbed in elevation. The sun felt more intense. Over the course of our drive, we had watched the corn shrink. Iowa's rain-fed crops were head-high and grass green. In the middle of Nebraska, stumpy stalks stood only knee-high in places and looked dry despite the watering. Now, in western Nebraska, corn crops fizzled altogether. Here began hardy wheat. And only some of the land was good enough for that. Most of the landscape was so rocky and dusty, barely pinned to the earth by low, hardscrabble weeds, that it could be used only as rangeland. We had come to my grandfather's home country.

Two hundred miles west of our campsite, where Nebraska's panhandle edged up to Wyoming, we arrived in Kimball. I knew my grandfather had grown up on a farm in Kimball County, but I had no idea how to find it. The county courthouse parking lot shimmered with heat, so Dan dropped me off and went looking for a shady place to park. I trudged up the cool marble steps inside the building, following signs for the assessor's office. Three women sat behind the counter: two young and one old. Each turned a brief eye from their work. Not recognizing me, they said nothing. "Hello," I smiled. "I was just hoping you might be able to help me figure out how to find the farm where my grandfather was raised."

"Do you have the parcel number?" one of the younger women asked.

"Just a name—my grandfather's dad."

"Well," said the other young woman, "with nothing but the name, the best we can do is let you dig around in the basement files."

Ever the romantic when it came to historical relics, I leaped at the chance to rifle through old records. "Just let me go find my husband, and I'll be right back."

As I scurried back into the office with Dan in tow, the old woman spoke up. "I was just telling these girls I'd probably know the farm," she said. "What was your great-grandfather's name?"

"Earl Ellis Hickman. My grandfather was Earl Lee Hickman."

The old woman let out a laugh. Her coworkers dipped their heads and smiled, as if to say they should have known.

"I'm Anita Larson," the old woman said, coming to the counter with her hand extended. "I knew all of the Hickmans. I know the farm. I live right next to it."

Anita showed us a plat map on the wall and traced directions with a strong forefinger. "First, sixteen miles west to Bushnell. Then take the main road north through town. It'll be two miles on blacktop, then three more on gravel. Turn west again on Road 44 and watch for the farm—it's the first one you'll see."

As we thanked Anita for her help, she waved away our gratitude. "Now, which Hickman did you say your grandfather was?"

"Earl Lee."

"Oh! The baby." Her voice dropped. "He was the one with all of the health problems, wasn't he?"

I asked what she remembered.

"Well, I just recall he was kind of, well, a puny young man. And he just had a horrible, horrible time with the heat. On a day like this"—she gestured out the window—"he just had to do anything he could to get cool. He'd just try to stay close to the ground, or on the floor of a vehicle—just the lowest he could get. Wherever he was, he'd just crouch down like a . . . well, it was just awful for him."

I sensed that Anita had stopped herself from comparing my grandfather to a cowering animal.

"Everybody knew Earl had lots of problems," she finished. "You do know he's buried here in Kimball, don't you? The cemetery is on the west side of town, and the Hickmans are on the far side of the cemetery."

As I thanked her, she had an afterthought. "You know, your family's old farmhouse is still standing. My grandson is renting it for the summer, and I'm sure you could stop by. Where are you staying tonight?"

"We're staying with my great-aunt Sadie, my grandfather's sister, just over the border in Pine Bluffs," I said.

Anita's smile widened again. "Sadie is my friend. Make sure you bring her when you come to the farm. I'll meet you there tomorrow at noon."

Kimball County Cemetery lay beyond the car dealerships, an abandoned motel, and the wrecking yard. It offered the only green grass in sight. Beyond the cemetery's twitching sprinklers, rocky pastureland stretched like acres of burlap. Dan pulled into the cemetery and trotted out of the car toward the directory at the center of all the tombstones. Flags snapped in the warm wind, and mourning doves sneaked sips from shallow sprinkler puddles.

"Bonnie, come look at this," Dan called. He took me to the back side of the directory and began counting the Hickmans. "Cora, Donald, Earl Ellis, Ellis, Joan, Josephine, Mildred . . ."

"His aunt," I chimed in. "His cousin, his dad, his brother, his sister, his mom, another sister . . ."

Dan looked at me, surprised. "Nice work," he said.

I had been studying. I didn't know if it mattered whether I knew all of my grandfather's aunts and uncles, sisters and brothers, nieces and nephews. But in my search for a link between his life and mine, I had been memorizing every detail I could find.

Dan pointed west. "He should be right over there. You walk. I'll go get the car."

He must have guessed I would want a moment alone to say hello to the grandfather who had died when I was a toddler, the man to whom my mother, and my grandmother, had always attributed the shambled years of their lives. I wondered if I would feel anything. After all, it would just be a stone, with a shrunken body somewhere deep below.

I saw a pair of thick, granite slabs, side by side. Etched headstones and an ivory vase between them marked my great-grandfather and my great-grandmother: Earl's parents.

EARL ELLIS HICKMAN
1888–1959

and

JOSEPHINE PAULINE HICKMAN
1893–1957

And then I saw him. A square stone, flat in the grass, directly at his mother's feet:

EARL LEE HICKMAN
SEPTEMBER 8, 1930–DECEMBER 2, 1979

I knelt and burrowed my hand into the grass above the spot where I guessed my grandfather's heart, or perhaps his head, might be. I half expected to feel a touch of heat rising from him, a low hum of electricity.

Earl in there, I prayed, *I feel you. A shriveled wisp, small to your bones. Do you know me? Are you even there? Your jawbone easy side swinging when you laughed, your deep sunbeaten eyes. What can you tell me, now that I have come?*

As Dan trudged up, I could see his face was starting to sunburn. He slowed to observe the graves, moving his eyes from my grandfather to my great-grandparents and on to my great-aunts and great-uncles.

I had told my mother very little—only that I was going to be passing through some of her childhood places. I pulled out my phone and dialed her at work.

"You won't believe where I am," I said.

"I know! The Greeley house! By the pond?"

"Not yet," I said. "I'm in Kimball, Nebraska. I'm standing next to your father's grave."

She went silent. I thought we might have lost our connection. Then I heard her swallow and say, "I have no idea why that made me cry."

She had been almost twenty-five years old—a year younger than I was that day in the Kimball Cemetery—when her father was buried.

"What did you think about the way they put him right at his mother's foot?" I asked.

"What?"

"You know, the way he's right there with her, as though she's keeping him tucked under her wing the way she did when he was little."

"Bonnie, I've never been there," she said.

"You didn't come to the burial?"

"No," she said. "We had a little service in Seattle, and then we sent him on the plane to Nebraska. His sisters wanted to take care of things."

I wanted to ask why no one had flown with him, but I suspected the answer was much too big for an afternoon phone call at the office—and much too complicated for my mother alone to explain.

When I hung up, I thought of my grandfather's brain, sparking madly in the years before he died. He had lost his grip, but he still believed mightily in his potential. I wondered what, if anything, physically remained of that brain. Did little fossils of his memories—his delight and his despair—still mark the casket beneath me?

Aunt Sadie, the only one of my grandfather's seven siblings still living, answered the door in Pine Bluffs with soft hellos. She brought us into her living room, where every knickknack and photo stood in perfect order. The house was so clean, it begged to be inspected for dust. Rosaries, crucifixes, and mounted Bible verses rested alongside photos of Sadie's late family: parents, seven brothers and sisters, two sons, and her husband of fifty-five years, who had died four months earlier. An even wider array of photos displayed her three living children, with their own spouses and kids—my second cousins. Songbirds decorated everything: flowerpots and picture frames, teacups and keepsake saucers mounted on the dining room wall. Twelve different bird species chirped from the wall clock. Every hour on the hour, when Dan and I perked up and looked around to locate the sudden bird in the room, Sadie broke into a laugh.

I hadn't explained the motive for my visit, so Sadie became quieter and quieter as I probed about her little brother Earl. Did she remember him suffering as a child? People saw him as weak, helpless—did she think this caused him to take on too much later in life, going way over his head in pipe dreams and debts and addictions? What happened in Greeley when he had to pack up his wife and children and run? Wasn't that right after his best friend Junior was found with a bullet through his head? Was Earl a good father? Why did he die so young?

The more I asked, the more watery Sadie's brown eyes became. She tapped her cloud of white hair, smoothed her eyebrows, and began a rhythmic nodding, saying, "I don't know . . . I just don't remember . . ." Then she disappeared into the basement to root out a box of family photographs. Soon, I had pictures spread all over the dining room table. I took careful snapshots of each one. Faced with images of my grandfather as a tiny boy, I felt shame for my brazen prying. The pictures told me what I should have already understood. He had been a real child, not a research subject.

When Earl Lee was in kindergarten, they took his picture with the class. He wore tiny wire-rimmed glasses. They slid down his flat little nose a hundred times a day. His thin-fingered hand, like a weightless bird, flew up again and again to right them.

When Earl Lee was in second grade, the photographer accidentally cut off the side of his face at the edge of the class photo. The boy's head pointed down and to the outside edge, in a posture of shame. His worried eyes rolled up to meet the camera, and his lips parted in the quiver of a cry.

When Earl Lee was twelve, the dentist presented him with a wonderful, precious torture: dentures top and bottom, fitting right in with his own six teeth. His new teeth rubbed his gums until they oozed blood. For months, he could take out his teeth and eat or leave them in and smile. Already a pale thing of skin and bones, Earl grew thinner and grinned.

"Climb in," Sadie said the next morning, cranking her car's engine and setting the air conditioner on high. We raced a freight train full of new cars as we left Pine Bluffs, heading eleven miles east into Nebraska to visit Bushnell. Passing the town's population sign—162—we pulled across the train tracks onto Main Street. On either side of us, sheets of plywood shuttered the windows of eighty-year-old buildings.

"That started out as a bank," Sadie said, pointing to a stout brick structure. "Later my sister Betty had her beauty shop there. And that was our church," she continued as we passed another empty shell.

Dan gasped. "Even the *bar* is boarded up."

The post office and a small white church seemed to be the only viable establishments in town. Many of the houses stood empty, too.

When we passed the two-story high school where Earl, Sadie, and their brothers and sisters graduated, we saw crumbling limestone, pigeons roosting in abandoned windowsills, and the rim of a basketball hoop, rusty and stretched into an *S*, pointing toward the dirt. I heard Dan murmur from the backseat, "I've never seen anything like it."

We pulled out the far side of town, following the main road north into the tallgrass. Two paved miles led to a missile silo—we would learn that the plains states are pocked with them—and three miles of gravel took us to the turn for the Hickman farm. In the distance rose a low hill, with just enough pitch to showcase white rocks arranged in a giant *H*.

Sunflowers blazed from the ditches, white crepe prickly poppies bloomed from spiny stalks, and paddles of cacti bunched in the fields. Nothing else showed green. The fields either shimmered with buttery wheat or lay bare and roasting. Even most of the Chinese elm trees, soldiering in a row up to the farmhouse, were dead. Their stark white branches shot like flames at the high blue sky.

Anita greeted us and introduced her grandson and his roommate.

"You can go in," said one of the college boys. "But it's kinda dirty in there."

I started to say "no matter" when Sadie snapped, "Well, how come?"

"We're guys, I guess," the boy stammered.

"You're supposed to keep it clean." Sadie pointed at a dead rabbit in the yard that had been lazily shot from the house. Flies buzzed over its clumped fur. "You guys need to clean this up."

"We were gonna take a load to the dump today," the boy said, his voice nearing a whine.

"Well, will you get it done?"

He nodded as Sadie marched past the white wooden house, headed for the barn. Crossing the yard behind her, my eyes hungrily searched decades of detritus: empty gas cans and rusted fuel barrels, carpets and black trash bags, piles of old lumber and bent brown nails. I saw plastic gallon bottles and glass jars, shingles and mud flaps from trucks. In the distant fields hunkered an abandoned combine, two tractors, and an old, plump-fendered pickup. Their once-bright green, red, and yellow paint jobs had given way to bumpy orange rust. At the corners of the farmyard, whitewashed buildings had weathered to silver. The chicken house had collapsed into flinders, and the brood house next to it had shifted from a rectangle into a parallelogram pointing across the fields, as if it fancied itself in a sailboat race.

Sadie poked her head through the low holes that had once been the brood house windows. She let out a sharp breath at the junk inside: a warped old desk fan sinking into the soil, a lard can filled with crumbling screws, two colossal snarls of pink twine.

"It is amazing how things get," she said briskly. "It was never like this. We kept things nice."

A killdeer cheered as it went tripping past.

I looked up at the barn, with its broad, peaked roof. It was dark brown, the color of creosote. Lifted by hot wind gusts, sheets of metal flapped and crashed on the roof. Swallows cheeped and careened, warning us away from their nests. We stepped carefully inside the barn, tiptoeing across sections of collapsed floor.

Sadie pointed out the stanchions where her father milked his cows, averting her eyes from the high-spun bird's nest threaded over a pair of old-fashioned machine goggles someone had left on the railing a generation ago.

"The barn's gone to pot," she said as we stepped back out into the blazing sun. "It used to be painted red. Can you imagine? Someone should pick up all this wood and put it in a pile and burn it. And tear down these buildings and burn them, too, if they're just going to fall down like this." She glanced at me. "Wouldn't you?"

I didn't dare admit that I thrilled at the sight of all that junk. Everything was an artifact, a clue; every nail, every brick, every splintered slab of wood was something my young grandfather might have touched. I pictured his hands on the rough-handled pitchfork in the corner of the barn, and his lanky body leaning in the shady doorway. I imagined his skin cells floating in the dusty air, part of the ecosystem there. I wanted to breathe deeply, to get close to anything he might have touched, used, loved.

Sadie was leading us to the house when Dan made an abrupt turn and strode back toward the barn. "What do you see?" I called.

"Something cool," he hollered back. "I just have to take a picture, then I'll meet you inside."

The house certainly reminded me of places I had seen during college. The boys had strewn beer cans inside and out. A dartboard was the only decoration on the living room walls. An array of couches, which seemed to double as beds, stuffed the core of the tiny three-bedroom dwelling. But Sadie managed to find vestiges of her childhood that made her smile. "My father made these cabinets by hand," she said in the kitchen. I wondered if those graceful built-ins had sparked my grandfather's passion for woodcrafts. I thought of the cedar chest, burl clock, and redwood table my mother had inherited.

"And look," Sadie went on. "Here are my mother's flour and

sugar bins. She baked all the time—bread, pies." Where things were missing, Sadie conjured them: "Over here was the pot-bellied stove. Our mother had the piano right here. Her arms went up and down, and she laughed when she played. She just bounced! And this is the room where we were all born."

As Sadie and Anita chatted, I wandered down to the cool cement cellar. *This*, I thought, *must have been one of Earl's safe places in the summer.* A little rodent lay bloated on the floor. I suspected Earl brought his books with him and exercised his brain when his body needed to rest.

As Sadie pulled the car back onto the highway, Dan passed me the digital camera with a picture on the screen. "Look what I found," he said. From the hayloft door, a metal basketball hoop cast a long shadow down the front of the barn. And wedged beneath it, a timeworn wooden plank sloped toward an imaginary free-throw shooter: It was an automatic rebound machine.

I had always known my grandfather loved basketball. Sadie had shown me pictures of my grandfather on the high school basketball team, though I knew that the higher Earl went in school, the more he struggled to keep up in the gym. He kept his jersey soaked in cold water even though he no longer shot hoops outdoors on hot days. By the time he graduated from high school, basketball was a memory for him, a hobby too strenuous to keep. Still, his tall sons—my uncles—played in high school and college. Basketball had always been a part of our family gatherings in Seattle—on TV during winter and in the backyard during summer.

It might have been natural, then, that I felt at home with Dan, the captain and star of our college basketball team. When I arrived as a freshman, he was a junior busy setting records for three-point shooting, free throws, and total career points. I fell quickly for his blue-black hair and long eyelashes, his gentle hazel eyes, the straight white teeth in his perfect smile. His easy

grins and bright laugh were contagious. Watching Dan play basketball was mesmerizing. He had found a way to play a frenetic
game with so much grace that at times I felt as if I were watching a ballet. Running drills, lifting weights, jogging to the gym
after dinner to shoot hundreds of free throws without missing—
all of it had come together to make him one of those athletes who
made everything look easy. Now he was twenty-eight, and I was
days away from turning twenty-six. We had been together for
eight years and married for one. My husband was still hitting the
bull's-eye, slipping the football between telephone wires and land-
ing soil-footed weeds in the yard bin like so many precisely struck
shuttlecocks. He loved to win, but more than that, he loved to
play. He had always said he wanted to start having children before
he was much older than thirty; he wanted healthy knees to play
sports with his kids—more than one, we both hoped—all the way
through their college years. But he knew our path to parenthood
might be thorny. Before we became engaged, he had asked me to
tell him more about Luke's condition; he knew it was hereditary. I
explained that there was a chance I carried the disorder.

"Is there anything they can do about it?" he had asked.

I told him that the gene mutation had recently been identified, so "they can pick out healthy embryos."

At the time, it was enough information for both of us.

Dan and I said goodbye to Sadie the next morning. I felt I had
botched my chance to learn from her by being too forward with
my questions. She had given me few details, but at least I now
carried images of my grandfather as a boy and deep impressions
of a hard landscape. The sun in western Nebraska was too intense,
the wind too dry, the storms too heavy. The baked earth resisted
cultivation, daring even the fittest men to wrest a living from it.
This was no place to be puny, I thought. *No place at all.*

"We were so, so happy in Greeley," my mother told me on the
phone as Dan and I drove across Wyoming into Colorado. I had

fallen into a pattern of calling her from the road to report the details I uncovered about her father and to ask any question that popped into my head. This time, I wanted her to give me the story of her family's rise and fall during their three years in Greeley, which ended in a sudden flight from town in 1962.

"Everything just fell apart," she said. "As soon as Junior died, it was like my dad became a different person. I never knew who he was after that."

Junior's death was the biggest turning point of my mother's childhood, and it had always carried an air of mystery.

"Do you remember Junior's last name?"

"Gronquist, I think," she said. Then, "Oh, my God. You have to tell me what you find out."

The Evans Cemetery, sitting at the edge of Greeley, was our first stop after hours of driving from Sadie's. We had plans to meet my grandfather's old friends, Jack and Mary Lewis. But first, I wanted to see if Junior had any secrets to tell.

"This has to be it," I said to Dan as we crossed the shady grave-yard. "His family said to look for a white military stone, right up next to the road." I had called his relatives from the phone book.

Junior had been born the same autumn as my grandfather, and like my grandfather, he had been tucked with his mother to rest.

JAY RAY GRONQUIST
OCTOBER 26, 1930–APRIL 24, 1962

On the day he died, Junior was thirty-one years old. My mother, the oldest of three children, was eight. The tulips were blooming. "I remember something weird I started to do," my mother told me. "I would walk around to the side of the house and make sure I was by myself. Then I would just stare into the tulips, all red and yellow, and I kept whispering to myself over and over again, 'When you die you never ever ever ever come back. When you die you never ever ever ever come back.'"

A warm, humid wind shuffled through town. Tall pines listed above us, sweeping bristled shadows across the cool headstones. I stared at Junior's marker, then shifted my eyes to the grass in front of it. I tried to see through the ground, to focus on the outline of his body. He felt much further away than my grandfather had.

"What happened to you?" I whispered. "Why did everything change when you died?"

I heard nothing in the wind and nothing from below. Was I on the right path? If my grandfather had something to do with Junior's death, why would that matter to me?

Later that afternoon, Jack and Mary greeted us at the door of their 1950s rambler, dressed almost exactly alike. They both sported plaid, short-sleeved, button-down shirts tucked into walking shorts. White athletic socks shot up their calves, and their white tennis shoes gleamed. Jack was short, sturdy, and bald, with smooth cheeks, a wide smile, and clear eyes. Mary was a bit taller, with gray hair beginning to turn white. She seemed less tired than her husband, and although she was happy to let him be the center of my interview, she seemed more certain about things.

"Your grandfather got to the top of things very fast," Jack said as we settled onto the couches in their white-carpeted living room. "Whatever he did, he learned very quickly."

I thought of my brother, who was the same way.

Jack continued. "It took no time at all for him to learn how to be a hospital orderly, how to drive an ambulance. Scientific terminology, medical procedures—you name it. He knew the chemical composition of every drug on the market. He was always cooking up ideas that someone should have thought of before. He thought grocery stores ought to have pharmacies inside. He figured there should be little convenience stores open all night long. And you know about his inventions, don't you?"

Perhaps because it was one of the few things for which my mom felt proud of her father, it had been one of her refrains as I grew up: "My dad was a genius, you know. An inventor." But I had never known what that meant. Did he help his kids make the best backyard forts in the neighborhood? Did he dream up bleeping robots that could cook and clean and do homework? Or did he really design and build contraptions, then go through all the legal steps to put them on the books? Did he invent for a *living*?

A few weeks before our visit to Greeley, I had visited Iowa's collection of patent volumes in Des Moines, a two-hour drive from our house. Dan had good-naturedly agreed to visit the city with me; we still felt new to the Midwest after our move from Seattle, and neither of us had seen the state capital. The city turned out to be dreary, particularly on that unseasonably grim spring day. No one walked the downtown streets, and cafés sat empty. But the library next to the capitol building was stately and ornate, with a whole wing devoted to the patent collection. As Dan explored the cluster of historic buildings around us, I began pulling red and brown volumes from the shelves: 1954, 1955, 1957. And soon I had a pile of photocopies on the table.

"I do know about his inventions," I answered Jack. "The humidifier, the foot rest, and we all know about the Nebulizer. He made a lot of money on that, didn't he? Enough to start making all of his other investments, right?"

"Oh, yes," Jack answered absently as he gazed at a handful of photos he had taken at Greeley General staff parties half a century before. He had pulled them from his collection to give to me. The images were crystal clear and rich with color; Jack had always been a photographer and had carefully developed the film himself.

"You look at these pictures," he said, pointing to a series taken in a wood-paneled room filled with attractive young nurses and doctors in their twenties. "Your grandfather was the center of attraction. Everybody liked Earl. Just look at the way people stared at him. It's admiration all the way—particularly the girls. And he was always willing to help anybody."

"Maybe too willing," Mary said, prodding Jack to explain.

"I always called it skimming," Jack said. "Once he started making money on that Nebulizer, he had his fingers in a lot of things—medicine, real estate, manufacturing. And it seemed like it didn't matter who he partnered up with. He was just too trusting. His partners would take advantage of him, skimming money off the top so nothing trickled down to him. And sooner or later he'd be aced out."

"By someone like Dr. Helman?" I asked. Mary nodded. I had heard Dr. Helman's name over the years, and he had always been painted as a man who began as a father figure to Earl only to eventually manipulate and take advantage of my grandfather. But common sense told me my grandfather could not have been a perfect innocent. The stories in my family were full of gaps, and I encouraged Jack and Mary, just as I did all of my grandfather's old friends as I met them, to tell me what they really thought. It wasn't personal to me, I insisted.

"That Helman," Jack said, shaking his head slowly. "That doctor had plenty of skeletons in his own closet."

"What do you mean?"

"You know I worked at the funeral home with your grandfather," Jack said. "And you know Helman was an anesthesiologist. Well, I buried at least one of his mistakes. A baby. It's not the mortuary's job to inform the family. It's the doctor's. To this day, the parents don't know what really happened. And there were more stories like that," Jack said, pressing his lips together as if to keep himself from revealing more.

"Do you remember Junior?" I asked. "My mom says her life was turned upside down the day he died. Do you know why?"

"There were some rumors. They bothered your grandfather tremendously. He was the lowest I'd ever seen him." Then Jack looked me right in the eye and said, "Your grandfather was a friend to everybody."

"Especially Junior," Mary said. "Junior was kind of a loner. He would have been by himself all the time if it weren't for your grandfather."

Jack stood up, smoothing the crinkles from his shorts. "Well?" he said. "Texas Barbecue?"

At the roadhouse an hour later, I was almost comatose, stuffed with salad, pulled pork, beans, applesauce, and corn bread. Mary had described the progress of her raspberry patch, and Jack had detailed Colorado's aviation history. But before the check could come, a small gang of servers hustled around the corner of our wooden booth, peanut shells crunching beneath their shoes. Dan beamed as our waitress set a candlelit brownie sundae on my place mat and began to sing.

"Happy birthday, Kiddo," he said.

I had turned twenty-six. A strange thought settled over me as I blew out the little flame. I had always said I wanted to have my first baby at twenty-eight. My mother had been twenty-four when I was born, my father twenty-five. As a child, I loved their youthfulness and energy. I felt proud in college when I had occasion to share that my parents were still enjoying their forties. Giving their kids the best years of their life, they showed us what it looked like to live and look forward to life all at the same time. Watching them freewheel through their late twenties, I sprinted through night-chilled grass during their boisterous beer-tasting parties and coed softball games; I danced when they danced. Because they didn't separate the fun years of their lives from responsibility, I learned it wasn't necessary for me to do this, either. Family and freedom could coexist—it was simply a matter of attitude. In high school, when a girlfriend asked me when I wanted to start having kids, I named my twenty-eighth year without pausing. It simply felt right and continued to do so as the pieces of my adult life—marriage, career, fertility—fell into place. Still, until the moment I faced my twenty-sixth birthday candle, motherhood had always seemed very far away.

We had planned to camp that night in a county park outside of Greeley, but my mother had another idea. "It's called the Sod Buster Inn," she said over the phone. "You're in the Colorado Room tonight. Happy birthday!"

I hadn't noticed the tension in my back until we stepped through the doorway of our room. A glance around made my shoulders relax. A king-size four-poster bed with a handmade quilt invited us to snuggle in early. Two velvety armchairs anchored the bordello red carpet. And in the very center of the room shone an enormous white claw-foot tub with glittering fixtures and a bottle of bubble bath.

After turning the water on, I pulled out the stack of my grandfather's legal records—titles, property transfers, promissory notes—that we had looked up earlier in the day. "Can you make any sense of these?" I asked Dan, plunking the pile on the bed.

I slid down into the tub until tiny bubbles snapped against my chin, soaking and listening to the rustle of pages. Every few minutes, Dan murmured with surprise. "Geez," he said, looking at the size of the debts my young grandfather had shouldered. "Oh, man." Records bearing my grandfather's name turned up one after another from the days immediately preceding Junior's death.

When I climbed into bed, my skin still prickled from the hot bath. Dan had fallen asleep as soon as he crawled beneath the sheets. I lay on my back with my eyes open. For weeks, I had been trying to picture my grandfather without the help of photographs. Most nights, especially back in Iowa where the events of his story felt so distant, I had been asking for dreams. I wanted him to be more than a foggy memory, filtered through his family and friends. I wanted Earl to stand in front of me so that I could feel the electricity of his nerves, smell the heat of his flesh. More than anything, I wanted him to speak. I wanted him to tell me what it felt like to live with his medical condition, and why he couldn't survive past forty-nine. I wanted him to tell me what had happened to Junior. I worried that without my grandfather's voice, without his specific guidance, I was in danger of misinterpreting him. Maybe he would tell me that I was focusing too much on the pain that he caused his family and friends—and not enough on the pain burbling in his organs. Or perhaps he would tell me that his transgressions were pure malignance, unrelated to his disorder. Or that HED did, in fact, shape his very sense of self, the weight of it warping every act of his adult life. Maybe he would tell me not, for any reason, to have a baby with the disorder. Maybe he would tell me to decide for myself; that every life begins untainted, despite lineage, despite flesh, despite the backward glances of parents.

When I switched off the lamp, my heart started to thump. I wasn't normally uneasy in the dark, but why couldn't I see anything? Not the windows, not the armchairs, not the bright white tub. Our charming room turned suddenly chilly. I felt strangers around me: ghosts breathing in the bubble-steamed air. I wanted to shut my mind to this, to take a night off from the eeriness. I wanted to think about my birthday, about candles, about light things. But something told me that now, more than ever, I needed to stay open. If these ghosts—Earl, Junior, perhaps others—wanted to find me, I had to let them. I breathed faster, slowly realizing that the strange black chill wasn't coming from the room. Something dark was emerging from me—something I needed to learn more about. I dropped into a black sleep filled with whispers, and I tried to listen.

earl

I couldn't breathe at night. I would wake up in a panic because I forgot to inhale. On summer nights in 1960, I would wake up before the sky could go all the way black. I would wake up later when the cats shrieked. Then I would wake up before sunrise to the sprinklers twitching. Then when the grass stretched in the first full rays. Exhausted. I needed something to comfort me so I could work, so I could provide for my family. I took Talwin, from my Winthrop sample case. My sweet little wife sighed, watching me swallow the pills: "Treat the cause, Earl. Treat the cause."

So I went under the knife, to have my septum straightened, to have my nose given just a little shape. A little less of a round, tiny, blunt end. More structure. The doctor said, "Hm, hmm— this should do you at least a little good, Earl." And how. Even if it didn't make me breathe better, at least I could breathe easier not meeting businessmen with my button nose.

Still, to improve matters, I started taking something before bed. The nose drops didn't work anymore. The syrups didn't work anymore. I could always take something to help me wake up in the morning, but one night I wondered, *Why not take something to sleep better in the first place?* I knew from the medical literature that with apnea like mine, the breathing would start up again by itself, and it wasn't necessary to wake up and restart respiration consciously. So, then: Nembutal at night, sometimes an upper in the morning, and Talwin in the daytime. My nose looked better. And I was breathing easier.

"Earl," my wife pleaded softly by my nightstand as I napped. "You seem so strange."

There were bottles now, not just sample packets.

"What are you doing with these pills? What doctor would give you all of these?"

In my moment between sleep and waking, when everything was possible and all forgiveness within reach, I heard myself release a single, ancient whimper.

"Oh, oh," my wife said, dropping to her knees to cup my face, her hands cooling my jaw. "I know, I know. I love you, too."

But then, that very evening: "Come out of there," she hissed against the door. "For God's sake. What are you doing? You did this at Joyce and Jim's, too. Can't you just stop it and come out and act decent?" She believed it was a matter of the will.

Dr. and Mrs. Helman had come for bridge. I knew it had been long, my spell in the bathroom. One thing was preparing the medicine, crushing the capsules. Then there was the wait, something to endure and then savor privately. I wanted to come out bright and shining.

"Paula, Greggy!" I heard her in the kitchen, calling out into the yard. "Time to get in here and clean up for bed. Where are you?" Her voice had gone to the patio while our guests waited at the card table. She was giving me time. My racing heart slowed. The kids could have been anywhere on the block, horsing with the neighbor kids, that pack of crazy dusk-time goblins.

And then her singsong, like a buttress: "Mrs. Helman, more wine? Doctor? Not for either of you? I'll just check Earl." My peace broke. I had been so happy alone. "Just a minute," I told her through the door, trying a soft singsong of my own. "I'll be right there. I'll just finish up."

I heard her say, back in the living room, "Well, how about some more almonds then?" and soon came the sound of nuts tumbling into the bowl. I flushed and exited, as if nothing had been strange, as if twenty minutes had not passed, as if it hadn't happened the last visit as well. As if there weren't a flush in my cheeks and a crease like sweet love at the corners of my eyes and a certain chemical joy in the corners of my mouth that nothing could unbend. Esta came in with the almonds, and the kids raced in behind her, nighttime trailing from their pores. Paula with her grass-green soles thumping the floor on her way to my lap. I had never seen a more darling thing.

"Hi, Baby Doll," I said, hugging her in. "You want to help Daddy play bridge?"

"Sure!" She was breathless, grabbing butter mints. "And Daddy?"

"Yes?"

"When you pick me up from kindergarten, can you wear a hat from now on?"

"Well sure, Baby Doll. But why?"

"Because you don't have any hair," my small daughter said, matter-of-fact, as if hats simply followed from baldness. Despite myself, the rubber smile fell down, and Esta saw this in a glance. In that moment, she knew that I would go back into the bathroom, to do my part to ameliorate the mood of the evening. She grabbed our daughter from my lap, marched her down the hall, planted her like a stick in her room, and shut the door hard. "Your daddy loves you!" she shot through the knob.

Esta tried for me. She held me as we slept. But she was fierce for the children.

"Earl, you have got to keep a lock on those Winthrop drugs downstairs. You put the latch on the closet but I keep finding the latch undone when I go down to run the laundry. You just imagine if the kids got into it. Kill them just like that."

She questioned me more and more.

"Listen to me," I said. "It's time to invest all that money from the Nebulizer—and there will be more. I trust Helman just fine. He has been with me since the beginning, and I owe him my loyalty. I'm going to quit Winthrop at the end of the year."

"No you don't," Esta said.

"Listen! You want me like Calhoun, driving the whole West with Winthrop and going madder and madder with no plan for anything else all his life? There are better things for us, Esta. Watch: '61 will be a dream. I'll be here with you and the kids. Helman and I are going to set up a medical building right in the center of Greeley. I'll drive up there a couple of times a week, but that'll be it. Imagine. It could be this way the rest of our lives: all of us together, all the time, the money just making itself out there. I just have to take out one small loan to get us started. The Nebulizer money will be flowing in soon, and I can pay back the loan. Helman's put in enough. And I do trust him. All right? So now look. Look how beautiful you look in that blue."

"Worrying makes me sick," she said. "You drive me crazy."

So I danced for her: "Greg! You're going to be a cowboy movie star! Paula! You'll be on the stage twirling! You can have anything you want! You can do anything you want!"

"Earl, for God's sake," Esta said, rolling her eyes, trying not to smile. "What are you talking about?"

"You'll see, Mommy!" I sang for her. "It's going to be like the movies! Our whole lives!"

But Esta was the one who had entertained that night, watching Helman's expressions, her ears sharp for the tone of his commentary, while I required my privacy in the bathroom. Esta knew he had begun to disdain me. She wanted me to prove myself, to make the doubters sorry. She would fight me and fight me, then finally hold my hand.

Junior came to our kitchen in Broomfield that winter, twice a week after work, 7:00 on the dot. I remember snow so quiet falling in the night, and Esta down the hall with the kids and a new one on the way. Junior said to me, "That's something, Earl. Good for you. This house and the growing family and plenty of investments and Esta. She's quite a woman, Earl."

"What do you mean there, Mister?" I teased him.

He was too easy to unnerve. "I only mean I just hope I can get a woman someday like her. But it doesn't look like I'll have a wife ever. Can't even find a girlfriend. But thanks for this coffee here, and thanks for being a friend, you know, with all the coffee you give me," he said, winking one eye fast, since we both knew it wasn't really coffee he came for, but samples from my locked closet.

"It's fine, you," I told him. "You just tell me whatever you need and I can get it for you, no problem. So what's this going on at work? Calhoun says they're hassling you?"

"I don't know, Earl." There was a strange shudder from him. "I just don't have a good feeling there. I don't know what the people think of me. They all seem antsy when they stand by my desk. They're fidgety all the time. And they're not even the ones with something to worry about. I'm the one. I can tell something bad is coming. Something bad. I think I got to get out of there, Earl."

There he was, good Junior, with the job of a lifetime at Dow Chemical and working on programs he could tell no one about, not even me, and he kept telling us that someone wanted to bother him. Someone wanted to get him.

"What do you mean, 'get you'?" I asked him once.

But his two eyes just waved to the side, and his head followed, and he dozed at the kitchen table because our "coffee" had done its trick.

Peaceful and nice, I thought, looking at his boy face.

In 1961, I did quit Winthrop. I had set up some pharmacies. Knowing the industry was growing, I set up a property in Greeley with Helman and one in Kimball with my brother and found pharmacists to set up shop. The summer before, on our visit to Alberta, Esta's parents had agreed to invest their life savings from the farm. I had come to believe in Hans, that jaw-set Estonian. He took his vodka straight and warm. His sweat rolled beneath all that wool as he worked. He never bent to modernity. I wanted him to stay that way: trousers hung from braces and shoes shined every Sunday. But I wanted him to have a stake, too. The world was changing right around him and his butter-cheeked wife, and still they hardly spoke English. I asked him in the machine shed, "Hans, tell me, do you have savings? Do you want me to invest it? Make the money grow? I have an idea." He unbent from the tractor, wiped black grease from his hands on a rag that surprised me, it was so white. By that evening, with Esta's help explaining, I convinced them that we would invest their money well and give them a better retirement than their $20,000 ever could. And still, just in case, Julene said to Hans, she had her egg money, which penny by penny had made a good account.

As we drove back to Colorado, I felt fine. I had twenty grand in my suitcase, and it made me feel benevolent, this responsibility I accepted. Saving these poor, simple folks from their tired, old ways. They could keep on living as they did, in sepia, and I would take care of them. What did they know? Baking pastry and milking cows. It would be Pertel Inc., their last name, and I imagined them imagining it: a company bearing their Estonian name in the United States of America. Surely they never could have dreamed.

Esta and I, we had dreamed. And now it was coming true. I surprised her and bought a lot on Glenmere Lake up in Greeley. Exactly across from the grass hill next to the water, where we sat on a picnic blanket before we were married. I expected glee from her, but "I know, I know," I found myself saying to her tears. "It's so perfect here in Broomfield. I know, with the lawns and the barbecues and our friends. But we can have the dream house now, on the lake, and I can be even closer to work. The house will be twice the size of this one. And we can do whatever you want with it. Fireplace, anything. We'll build it brand-new and you can have all of your choices, all right? Colors and rooms and the yard—we can do it all to our taste. And the little lake and the ducks right there for the kids, and ice skating in the winter? Esta? Think of having the new little one and how much more comfortable we'll all be."

She straightened up for the kids. We told the kids they were the luckiest kids in the world, moving to Greeley right by the lake.

"We think Tommy and Gary are the luckiest kids," Paula said of the boys next door.

"Why?" Esta asked.

"Because their dad rides them on his handlebars wherever they want on Saturdays," Greg said.

"All our dad does is sleep on the couch," Paula said.

"Yeah," Greg said.

"Your dad loves you," Esta said, warning them.

I said nothing. They would see.

I took to driving around Greeley in the late afternoons, to survey my holdings and watch the progress of the house.

"I know what you're doing," Esta said, startling me on a windy day as I stepped out with the car keys. "I can picture it exactly. You show up at these pharmacies and you tell these poor idiot clerks who know no better that you're just there to check on some inventory, and you use those snake fingers of yours to slip the pills home. And now you've got Junior doing this garbage, too."

"That's crazy," I said, tongue dry. Somehow hearing her say it made it sound like stealing.

"Earl," she whispered. Her urgency was changed, enticing. "I read something in my magazine. Can you tell me something? I have a question—I've been wondering. What can you say about these diet pills? Do they work?"

As the weeks went by, I could see the pills made her feel fine and sunny in the mirror. She watched me watching her, and both of us felt for the moment safe and daring.

"Let's take the whole gang to Barons with us this summer," she said with spring sun in her eyes one morning. "Calhoun and Betsy can bring the kids. Junior can meet my sister Wilma. We'll make it a real big time."

How could I not agree to this? But I dreaded returning to her parents' farm. Their money had been quickly swallowed. I could take out more loans, of course, to pay them back, to tide them until their last days. I would do what I had to do. But I knew when we got there, Esta would make me update them.

"Come on, kids, what do you think?" Esta asked them. "Let's go this summer up to the farm! We'll ride in Dad's new car all the way there and see Grandma and Grandpa and sweet Aunt Wilma and Blackie the bull and the chickens and the hay bale mountains and the windmill and all that wheat!"

We had only been a few hours out of the car that July, our bodies barely unbent from the long drive, our eyes adjusting to evening, when Esta put the last of our clothes in the dresser and said, "Mum and Dad will ask me about that money they put in. The pharmacy. Don't you have some interest to pay them, some sales or profit or whatever?"

My answer surprised us both. My body lurched from the bed and out the side door, where I vomited blood into the dirt. Esta's eyes were wide and wet, her pretty lips closed. She got her mother's spade and scraped at the ground, covering the thick black puddle I had made. In the morning, the chickens pecked there.

All I could do was show my goodwill. I climbed up the windmill in the early day, tried to straighten that one pesky blade.
Paula stood in her bare feet below. Between clanks of the wrench
as I struck metal, she screamed up, terrified, "Daddy! Don't fall!
You'll die!"

On the last day of our trip, I did the sort of thing I thought
I would never do. At the bank, "Yes, sir, my mother-in-law. You
know her—nice lady, doesn't speak English, just Estonian. Yep,
Julene Pertel, shy thing, all right. She asked me to come with-
draw the money in her egg account. Ha-ha, yeah, she calls it her
egg account—it's saved from selling the chicken eggs. Yes, cer-
tainly. My name's Earl Hickman, her daughter Esta is my wife.
No problem at all, sir. Here is the account number. That's right.
Fifteen hundred it is, then. Thank you, sir—enjoy the afternoon.
Feels cooler out now, doesn't it?"

And a few hours later we drove. Smooth like river water that
night, as we whistled down the fields. My wife holding our new
baby, another strong boy, and my back pocket bulging. "Sleep,
sleep," I whispered to the kids in back. "Sleep, sleep."

In Greeley I was on top of the world. My afternoon drives were
other people's coffee break or shoulder rub or pleasing bank
statement in the mail. Sunny and all the naked trees shivering
under a little wind, but warm and sweet in my car. North to the
bowling alley called Classic Lanes: mine. A few blocks west to
the Sundown Motel: mine. The café across the street: mine. The
two little one-story houses downtown: mine. The medical center
full of tenants: mine. Hoffman's liquor store: mine. Pharmacies
in Greeley and in Casper and in Kimball, too: mine.

Esta always said, "*Percentage* yours, Earl. Not yours; *percentage* yours."

"My wife too proud to show it," I told her back. She came
home with dresses for her, dresses for Paula, smart new coats
for all of us.

I drove down and took another look at the warehouse for lease on Eighth, and I decided that would be it. It was just right for the new operation: mine.

Junior still came by. Now to our new table in Greeley, twice a week after dinner, while Esta was busy with the kids and their toothbrushing and pajamas on the other side of the house.

"Say, Junior, listen," I told him just before New Year's. "I've got something I want to tell you about. Here's your coffee," I winked. "You tell me what you think of this idea, all right? This chemist I met has a formula for a powdered enzyme. You shake it down the drain or the toilet or wherever there's a clog of some kind, and the enzyme eats right through it. But it's all natural and biodegradable and not even poisonous if the kids get into it. Although it's got quite a stench, so I can't imagine anyone trying a taste. Anyway, I'm calling it Enz-All. What do you think of that? *Enz* as in *enzyme*. This stuff is good for large spills in a place like a hospital or a restaurant, but also every housewife will want a small canister in her cleaning supplies. I'm taking it to the shelves. Safeway stores have already agreed to give it a run. I've got people lined up to print the packaging I designed, and I've got distributors on board. And now I need a right-hand man. A guy like you, Junior. A guy I can trust."

His small eyes had been so dull in recent months. But now I saw a spark.

"Tell me, Junior," I asked him after a moment. "How much money do you have saved?"

He stiffened.

"You'll make it all back, times ten, in a year or less," I said. "Just think about it. And take it easy there at Dow. You have other options, all right? Look at all that money you have, just sitting there. You really ought to invest it. There'll be lots more coming. Believe me."

He could see I was certain.

Still, Esta tugged against my hopes. "Earl, what are you doing?

What are you thinking taking out another loan from a friend? And from the bank in Casper, too! Oh, you think you can hide it. These guys know you have nothing. Big Earl. Always pretending. Everyone sees right through you. Sure, and we all know what's next. Go ahead. Just go in the bathroom and do your little garbage and then go to sleep on the couch. Do it."

All I could do was press on. The money was so close. Always right there, just behind one or two last things that had to go right.

"Junior, here," I told him at my table. "I got these business cards printed up for you. We can start work tomorrow down at the warehouse. It's still full of onions drying out, but I leased it starting now, so we can get our office in order and start bringing in our stock."

It was something to see him so proud, flipping through his Enz-All cards. They were all the same, but he wanted to look at every single one. He was tired of being a yes-man for Dow. So he quit right after New Year's Day and came to work with me. We each had a desk in the office in the middle of the warehouse. I told him, "First, we got to get our capital together. So Hoffman's got to get me those late rents for the liquor store, and we need to come up with another few thousand, and this Enz-All is going to take right off. What do you think? You have some thoughts on that?"

"I could put in," he said. His eyes stayed away from mine.

"Right. So you said you have a certain amount of cash. Do you have that precise amount still?"

He nodded. I wondered if he was going to weep.

"Trust me, Junior, all right?"

At the time, things weren't going as well as Dr. Helman hoped with our little corporation. He embarrassed me rotten in those weeks. "Earl, you're stealing our assets. You're taking pills from our pharmacy like a lunatic, slurping them down night and day, and you sleep through our meetings. I should buy you out. You bring in nothing anyway, you're so busy with this Enz-All project and whatever else."

He left me speechless, going on in his fit.

"You're overextended, man. Just think about it."

But I wasn't. He just didn't know. He wanted what I had, that was all. So I told him, "Sorry, Doc. My shares aren't for sale."

He said, "You need your head checked."

But Junior and I could work into the nights without fighting like that. He would plod in his way. I would tell him where we were sparking, where the numbers were good. We typed up letters like mad to distributors. The warehouse had no more onions, and the shelves were stocked with Enz-All now, eight-ounce cans and one-pound cans. We even had Enz-All in tablet form, with our own custom dial-a-pack, a plastic rotary case with a hole in the bottom for the tablets to drop out one at a time. Once a day into the toilet for better plumbing health.

She asked every night, as if my answer could change, "Earl, are you coming home for dinner?"

"Don't I always?"

"Yes, but are you *staying* home after dinner, and will you read your kids a book and play with the baby and come to bed with me? Or are you going to crawl in late again, looking like a skinny, old ghost and breathing in that awful, slow way?"

At times I couldn't hear her. Some of her words were just too hard; they glanced off.

"I'll see you at dinner," I said. "I love you."

And that night, late under my green lampshade, it was dark and quiet. From time to time I would hear one of my kids or my little angry wife taking one of those fast, scared breaths in sleep. I tried to concentrate on my accounting. *Columns. Here's what I need to add up. What's what. Focus. Columns on the page. It's money I owe to all my creditors, here. Would be good to consolidate: Make a bank loan instead, pay back individuals. So then: Repay full debt to Helman and my brother and the pharmacies. I owe. I owe them terribly. Stop taking the Talwin. But stop taking the heavy Talwin, keep borrowing small doses instead? To taper off. So, out proper remuneration also to Jim and Joyce, to Calhoun and Betsy, and the others. The numbers are clear, certainly, blue and running off the page . . . what happened to straight columns? Those straightedges were handy, weren't they? Remember those. Owl out there. Jump right out of my skin. Esta's parents and Junior, they can wait a bit longer than the others. There's more understanding there. But even so, this mess. These blue columns look like . . . could be. Might be. But I won't say "trouble" yet. Times of trouble, that's when God comes running down the skies. But does he come to giveth or to taketh away? No, focus. Bring the numbers down, come braiding down the page like a dance, wispy blue smoke dance after the sun goes down.*

I couldn't give up. I picked up the phone. "Junior? Are you awake? Can you meet me? Oh. Okay. Tomorrow then. But tomorrow night could be long, all right?"

And hardly anything could be accomplished before there was Helman again, telling me I couldn't even enter my own pharmacy holding, named after my own wife's parents. As if he thought he was my father: "You're cut off. No more. If the pharmacist sees you, he's to call me. If he can't reach me, he's to call the police."

I was perfectly honest with Helman, and I told him, "Look, here's my situation. I admit I haven't been my usual productive self lately. But I wasn't well. You understand? I'm getting better."

He just snarled his lip and said, "Go steal from your other pharmacies then. I don't care if they're a state away. You and your pathetic pants. Don't you see your pants are much too big?"

I no longer had the Winthrop samples. I could no longer enter my pharmacies. I had little to offer Junior. The money hadn't started coming in yet. And now he came to work glass-eyed and itching. One afternoon, Junior was late. Esta called me at the warehouse. "Betsy called. Junior drove all the way up to Cheyenne to get samples from Calhoun." At first my wife's shaking voice sounded angry. But then I heard sadness. "But Calhoun wasn't home today. He was out on the road. Betsy said that quiet old Junior pounded and pounded the front door and screamed at her little daughter Ellen, 'Let me in! You *let* me in!' and Ellen cried and cried. Betsy grabbed her and took her into the bedroom closet and the two of them stayed there in the dark until he was gone."

It could have been said that I did that to Junior. And to Betsy and that little girl of all people, that pale-faced poor little girl. But after all, Junior was a man, and he'd gotten himself into things, and he had to get out on his own, just like I did. Off the drugs and into the work, into the business, making the money. We were so damn close.

But Junior was descending somewhere. On Easter morning when he came for brunch, I met him with Esta at the door. "Hello, Esta," he said. And no greeting for me. I thought it was a joke, until I saw his face like stone. When everyone sat around the table, I stepped back from the feast with the camera. In the frame I got Paula in the background and my wife on one side of the table and Junior on the other side, and my God, something happened. I felt a chill down my belly. When the shutter snapped, I saw his eyelids come down half closed. His pupils were shiny as steel, flinting hard as winter right through me.

It was a quiet meal, and I tested as he went out the door. "See you at the office, all right, guy? See you there in the morning?"

He raised his eyebrow in a way I didn't recognize.

"A day off?" I asked. "All right. I hadn't thought of that, but I can work tomorrow and you rest. That's right—you deserve it. Happy Easter. Thanks for coming over, and you're a real fine friend, you know."

And so the next evening I worked late. That side of Greeley

was the part called Garden City, where alcohol was allowed. All the bars rowed up one beside the next. It was the night after Easter, such an innocent time, but there were all the drunks staggering out onto the street, reliable as winter.

Without Junior there that night, and without the light of day, it was heavy and dark. The orange and yellow Enz-All labels looked sickly to me, dreary as dead leaves. The papers on my desk confused me as the night went on too long. My ears kept straining for a familiar sound, and my mind was not writing letters, and my tongue was not licking envelopes. My ears searched, but everything was unfamiliar—the sounds of those lurchers, those bald corpses, those old men lost and fragile as tumbleweed. It was too late for more. Good to slip the key and shut it all behind me and suddenly remember: I had a *wife* at home under the cotton covers and three fluff-haired kids! I had to remember!

At home, the windows were all open and baby frogs sang out the spring. *For heaven's sake, imagine,* I heard myself think, *I almost missed it—I have to remember springtime.* A fresh gratitude swelled. There was my baby boy, sleeping with his round eyes gentled and his cheeks so narrow. And my bigger boy smelling of an afternoon: wind and grass and leaves sweetly rotting after winter's freeze. He had begun to smell like something other than a child. Sweet, clean, earth. And there was my girl in her room—my baby doll. It was black in her room; her night-light was burnt out again. I supposed she was having more of her bad dreams. I sat there on the edge of her bed, by her face, and searched the dark for her little head. I found her cheek, bright and shiny even in sleep, and I bent down to kiss her. But her skin was hard and cold, and I leaped away, my breath charging—"Paula! Oh my God!" I slammed the light switch to face my first dead child.

A moment later I found my daughter warm in bed with her mother.

"What is it?" Esta asked, hearing my heaving.

"Listen, Paula, wake up! Never do that again. You scared me. Don't put that big doll in your bed ever again. I thought it was you. I thought you were dead."

She cried, but rightly so.

By the next evening, I was changed. I knew now that everything before me was momentary. A blink's fortune. Any of it could change. Nothing would wait.

"Esta, you're sweet for the supper. What a pretty pink evening, isn't it? Greg? Paula? What are you going to do tonight? You can watch TV, you can go outside. What about the ducks on the lake? You kids are such great kids. You know, as soon as Daddy and Junior finish all this work, I'll be home here with you, and we can play and play."

"Oh, Earl, don't make too many promises," Esta said, and it smarted.

I drove down to the warehouse, stunned by the sky: a wild pink brimming in wheel rims and flashing in store windows. Either it was the loveliest night or I hadn't been on the lookout for loveliness, because here it was. My daughter alive and my happy sons. My proud wife. The blossoms opening around our front porch. Even baby ducks on the lawn, for Pete's sake.

It was so simple suddenly. The sweet small things. I told myself, *You cannot lose them.*

"Junior, say, isn't it a peaceful night?"

A nod from my friend, who seemed a little better.

"And listen, I know I promised to work late with you, but I'm going home early this time. Last night I thought my girl was dead, and I realized I ought to be home with my family a bit more. But when I said so to Esta tonight, she called me a liar. I'd like to prove it. Can we set you up with a few pages to type and a few calls to make? And can you stay here a bit later into the dark, after I leave?"

Another nod. But then I saw his eyes, wide open and frozen. I knew then: He believed we would fail.

"It's all going to be fine," I said.

His quaking face.

"I'm certain," I said.

It had been too long. There would be no sheriff's report of Junior's shooting, particularly if it had been classified a suicide. Without a police report, I would have too much to guess about what really happened between Junior and my grandfather. After a big breakfast at the Sod Buster, Dan and I prepared to leave town, assuming we had found everything there was to learn. But then I realized that a coroner's report on Junior's death might still exist.

I hopped out of the car in front of the coroner's tiny downtown office while Dan drove down the street to park. The office seemed no larger than a couple of bedrooms, so I assumed that Junior's file, if it existed at all, would be in a hard-to-locate storage container somewhere else in the county. But I was surprised. Just as Dan walked in, the chief deputy coroner, Tom Shimp, emerged from a back room and handed me a file marked with Junior's name. Beneath the certificate of death lay a brief coroner's report: "Gunshot wound to right temple—Suicide." It was a single page, with short comments penned into blanks. By comparison, Shimp showed us what a modern-day Weld County coroner's file looks like. On his desk sat the packet for a baby who had recently died mysteriously, exhibiting bruising up and down his back. The red file folder was stuffed two inches thick. "This is only his medical history," Shimp said. "We haven't even put in our report yet. This'll get a lot thicker."

I turned back to the single page about Junior. His body had been discovered in the morning on Wednesday, April 25, 1962, and the coroner determined that the shooting had occurred around 11:15 the night before, two days after Easter Sunday.

In wavering penmanship, the coroner noted that it was a housepainter named Sam McKinney who found the body. McKinney had been at work on a fence at the building's south side. Then he went around to the north side with his steel brush. Taking a break, he laid his brush in a high windowsill. When he went to retrieve it, his eyes flashed into the building, and there he saw the body.

Ralph Marcellus, the son of P. E. Marcellus, who owned the warehouse my grandfather leased, later insisted to me over the phone that it was in fact his father who had discovered Junior's body. "He walked in there to see how things were going because he hadn't seen rent in a while. He called out the fella's name— your grandfather's, I take it—and no one answered, so he went through to the back, and there was the dead man on the floor. So he went next door to get Gus Sherman from the farm machine shop, so there would be two of them when the police came."

The Marcellus family always supposed the dead man had just gone through a bad breakup with his missus, Ralph told me. But I knew Junior had no missus.

Rick Gronquist, Junior's close-in-age nephew, told me in an interview that the suicide determination had never made sense to his family. The bullet wound had been to the left temple, they all thought, and Junior was right-handed. But the coroner's report clearly stated that the bullet entered the right temple.

In a different conversation, Art Gronquist, Junior's brother, told me that no one in the family believed it was suicide, because the gun was discovered lying in Junior's right hand. Only a killer would place the gun in a victim's hand, trying to suggest that the wound was self-inflicted. A man having shot himself wouldn't think to hold on.

Even though she recalled awakening Earl herself with the news that Junior was dead, shot in the head, my grandmother also held an image in her memory of my grandfather walking into the warehouse that Wednesday morning: She could see her young husband stopping in his tracks, stunned at the sight of his friend on the floor, pale, motionless, and covered in blood.

Somehow, even my mother, who had been asleep in her bed at the time, recalled Junior's dead body: a man on his back, arms and legs akimbo, eyes closed, no blood.

None of these people ever saw the crime scene, though, or photographs of it.

Shimp handed me two grimed-over Polaroids. Fingerprints had leached away the color in the pictures, leaving whorls of tiny yellow lines where parts of the images should have been. One photo was taken from a distance. Junior's body rested on the warehouse floor, head at the left, feet at the right, face turned away from the camera. Double doors filled the frame behind a stocky body with a plump stomach. Junior appeared sockless in his loafers. Blood, black as ink, stained the floor around his head.

The second photo was only slightly clearer: a close-up, taken from directly above the body. I wondered morbidly if the photographer had to stand astride the corpse to take such a direct photo of the torso. Junior's arms lay to his sides like wings just opening: wrists bent outward, fingers pursed inward. One side of his button-up shirt was pulled loose from his belted jeans, revealing the smooth, white bulge of his abdomen and the very top of his hip bone. His head was wrenched to the side, showing the round, velvet entry wound at his right temple. Two wide ribbons of dry blood traced paths from the wound, bold as war paint. Both paths appeared to have traveled uphill, away from the wound, over the forehead and down again, over the face. One passed above the eye, then over the bridge of the nose. The other passed below the eye, finding its way down along the nose, crawling past the nostrils, and disappearing into shadow. I asked Shimp what he thought about the fact that the blood needed to have flowed uphill for it to have dried this way. He shrugged. "I see your point, but you never really know what the body does between the time a bullet enters it and the time it finally quits moving. Someone certainly could have positioned the body this way, or it could have moved involuntarily, shortly after he died."

The most remarkable thing in the photograph was this: a pistol resting high on Junior's chest, with the hammer tucked beneath his chin and the barrel pointing down his left arm. Could he really have committed suicide and ended up with the gun on his chest?

"That," Shimp said, "is impossible." Had Junior shot himself, especially from a standing position, the weapon would have ended up somewhere on the floor, he explained. Most likely somewhere off to his right side, down by his legs.

"But then again," Shimp said, "police practices being what they were back then, could be someone just picked up the gun and stuck it there to fit everything into the picture."

paula

I was eight years old when Junior died. That morning the phone rang, and I heard my mom say "What? Where?" and she started crying and didn't stop all morning. She ran in to wake up Dad and tell him. Greg and I were just trying not to be any trouble. But we wanted to know what happened. Mom said, "Junior died." We made our cereal, and I remember it seemed so loud falling into the bowl. I wanted to hear everything my mom and dad were saying. They were yelling in whispers. My mom said, "Well, how do we know it was suicide? How do we know someone else didn't do this?" and my dad said, "Because he had the gun in his hand."

Greg and I got dressed, and when it was time for us to go, my mom was standing in the hallway still crying, holding Curt, who was also crying, and my dad was visibly upset, but he wasn't crying. On the way to school, I said, "Greg, what's suicide?"

Greg said, "That's when you blow your brains out."

I had never seen gory movies or anything like that. My image was of Junior lying on the ground like he was asleep, holding a gun. All day I tried to imagine what it looked like when your brains were blown out. That afternoon I came home, and I said to my mom, "Greg said Junior blew his brains out," and that's when she finally looked at me. Maybe she was going to hug me. But the phone rang. It was her mother calling all the way from Barons, Alberta. It was so loud that my mom held the phone away from her ear. My grandmother's voice was hoarse but strong: "*Mind rööviti! Kus on muna raha?*" I've been robbed! Where is the egg money? "*Teie abikaasa*," she hissed. Your husband. My mom had been crying the whole day, and now she cried so hard she couldn't say anything to my grandma. My grandma just thought my mom felt bad about the missing egg money. She didn't know anything about Junior.

After dinner, my dad was sitting really quietly in the living room, at the window in his blue chair. My mom kept telling me and Greg not to get too close to him. But Greg kept taking one step closer and one step closer, really quietly, trying to see our dad's face. He turned back and looked at my mom and me standing there in the hall, and he said, "Mom, what's wrong with him?"

She said, "He's just very sad. His best friend died today."

Junior had been so weird when he came over for Easter brunch a couple days before he died. We didn't really like it in those days when he came over because my mom would talk in a different voice, which signaled to us that we had to be different, too. On Easter, for the only time I can remember, my dad told Greg and me that we had to be quiet and could not speak unless we were spoken to. It seemed like it was all about impressing Junior, and that Easter was all for him and not about us kids. I couldn't wait for the meal to be over. We just wanted him to leave. My mom was acting even more chirpy than usual. But I saw her wrists wobbling when she passed the scalloped potatoes.

I had heard them together that morning—my mom yelling at my dad, saying "Another loan, Earl? You're insane! Well, of course we have to pay the bills, but what about the ones after and the ones after?" I was always hanging around corners, listening. Half

the time I couldn't hear what my dad said. His voice was so soft
and gravelly, especially when he was tired. "Let's just forget it,"
she said to him. "It's Easter and we have to get everything ready.
Get these eggs and hide them around for the kids, will you?"

She came out and said to me, "When Junior comes over, be
good. Be real good." She practically poked her nails through my
Easter sweater. "Listen, Paula, I'm serious. Don't be loud and
don't show off and don't bother Junior. We can't make Junior
mad, all right?"

I asked her, "Why's Junior gonna get mad?"

She gave me a warning look and said, "I have to get in there
and devil the eggs. Go and tell your brother what I said."

A few days before Easter, my mom had told my dad she was sick
and tired of him working late every night, and she was going to
take Curt for an evening and go see Dr. Montgomery and his
wife. They used to play cards with the Montgomerys, but my dad
had gotten so busy. He wasn't really very social with their friends
anymore. I leaned in the car window while my mom put Curt on
the floor next to her. She just kept mumbling: "'After the work.
After the work.' It's all he ever says. It's nonsense. It's boggling.
Curty Curty Curt," she said to my little brother. "You little small
thing. You come with me. I might tell Mrs. Montgomery. I might
tell her I'm afraid. Earl's so strange. Maybe Dr. Montgomery will
know something to do. They love us, don't they? It's so hard to
tell anymore. Who is a friend? Who is a creditor? Who wants
Earl's money? Whose money does Earl want? I don't think he's
hit up the Montgomerys yet. I can tell them everything. They'll
answer from their hearts. Paula, go inside. Your dad is finally taking
some time off to play with you and Greg."

But instead my dad put us in his car and took us to the warehouse. It smelled like onions.

"Quit saying that," Dad said to us, so we quit saying it. But
it did smell.

Junior was sitting in the back office, and my dad went right in to see him. He said, "You two kids go play. Stay out of here— stay out of the office." But I barely moved because I wanted to see. Junior was talking fast, and he sounded scared. I saw my dad put his hand on Junior and tell him, "It's all going to be fine, just fine." He patted Junior on the shoulder, *pat pat pat.* I kept thinking how nice that seemed. Later that night, after Dad took us home to bed, I put up a fuss. I kept saying *Dad, Dad,* fast and scared as Junior had said *Earl, Earl* in the warehouse. I wanted my dad to pat me like that. Or tickle my back. Something to help me calm down.

But my dad just stood there in the doorway with the light behind him. He was a black shadow. He said, "Paula, please, shush. I'm very busy, all right? You have got to go to sleep now. Your mom will be back soon."

The day Junior died, Mom put Curt in the car and went to see the Montgomerys again. I don't even know if my dad knew she left. He seemed so far away, sitting there staring out the window and not saying anything. Greg and I just put ourselves to bed.

The next morning, my dad had to meet with the police at the warehouse. We were at home, and someone knocked on our door. "Go back to your room," my mom said when she saw me get up. "Just for a few minutes."

They knocked again, and I stayed long enough to see that it was Dr. Montgomery. He took off his hat and said, "Hello, Esta. How are you holding up?"

My mom said, "I'm quite fine, Doctor, and yourself? Coffee for you?"

She turned and gave me a look, so I went farther down the hall.

"No, Esta, please. Listen here," Dr. Montgomery stopped, as if he was waiting to see if anyone else was going to come into the room. Then he said more quietly, "I have to ask you a serious question. Where was Earl on Tuesday night? Could he have done this? Killed Junior?"

"I'll be honest," my mom said. "Earl came in for dinner and went out again. He does this every night. When he came home the kids were just to bed, and I was undressing. So he was here, and he went out, and he was back again, just like every night. Do I think he could have done this to Junior? For heaven's sake, Doctor. I really think more of Earl than that."

Later, we were all just sitting there in the living room. Greg was watching TV, and I was watching TV plus my mom's face and my dad's face. He was back from seeing the police and just sitting in that chair again. My mom had her hands in her lap and kept fidgeting. I heard my mom say, "Watch out, Earl." It was quiet, as though she wasn't sure she even wanted him to hear her.

He looked out the window. "It's just the Montgomerys."

She said nothing.

Then the doorbell rang, and Mrs. Montgomery came in first, and Dr. Montgomery came in behind her, for the second time that day.

The doctor shook my dad's hand but was looking at my mom, and he looked miserable. Dr. Montgomery said to my mom, "Earl needs a rest."

At first my dad looked happy, as if he thought it was a surprise. But then Dr. Montgomery put his hand low on my dad's back and kind of pushed him to the car. My mom came out with a little suitcase and passed it to my dad. He looked at her in shock. She came right back inside and poured tea for Mrs. Montgomery. Then she just sat on the couch and ignored me and ignored Mrs. Montgomery. She stared at her dress. I couldn't tell if she was mad or sad.

Mrs. Montgomery went over and patted my mom's hand. "You did the right thing, Esta. My husband is a good doctor, and he knows what's best. You're right to trust him. Earl's going to be fine. We're just as worried about him as you are. Mount Airy is a modern psychiatric facility, and it's just a short drive into Denver, and Dr. Montgomery got Earl signed on with their very best psychiatrist, Dr. Franklin Ebaugh—have you heard of him?"

"No, I hadn't," my mom said, trying to be chirpy again.

"Oh, Esta," Mrs. Montgomery said. "This is going to be good for Earl. They can cure him. Electroshock therapy is proven. He can stop with his habits, and the depression will end. Esta, dear. Look at me. If Junior killed himself, then Earl could be next. I mean honestly, had you seen those two lately?"

My mom didn't say anything then.

Mrs. Montgomery took a sip of tea that barely wetted her lipstick. "And, if Junior didn't kill himself," she said, "well, then Earl has some forgetting to do."

We left Greeley and returned to Iowa with as many questions as answers. For the rest of the year, I continued to explore places from my mother's childhood: other parts of Colorado, Nebraska, and Wyoming, and even my grandmother's childhood farm in Alberta. I flew to Seattle to sift through family artifacts, to interview my mother and my grandmother Esta at the same table, to ask them to tell and retell the stories that, in one way or another, opened into my own. My grandmother pulled out stacks of photographs for me. Her sister mailed more from Canada. Into my suitcase, my mother piled her old letters and poems and artifacts in crumbling envelopes. Uncle Greg, usually upbeat and self-assured, told stories with his eyes hidden. Dan asked questions. I had dreams. It seemed each person in the family held a few pieces of the larger story and welcomed the chance to unburden themselves. They routed every last scrap my way—here, a fur coat; there, a family Bible; here, too, a movie ticket stub, a photo of that haircut, and this, Earl's cane, the bone handle so soft. Parcels arrived in the mail: from Jack and Mary, a rectangular tin of Enz-All, shaped like an old cocoa can; from Colorado, the life story of the famous psychiatrist who oversaw

Earl's mind-altering electroshock therapy after Junior's death; from the Wyoming State Historical Society, jail records from my grandfather's confinement for fraud two years later.

I carefully opened my suitcase and packages, sifting, considering. I felt my family members—perhaps even my ancestors— watching and waiting, each clutching their own prayer, as I pulled all the fragments together and held them up to the light.

part three

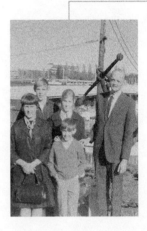

The Hickman family (*clockwise*):
Esta, Greg, Paula, Earl, and Curt
in Seattle, Washington, 1969

Outside the bungalow, the giant quince bloomed coral. White tulip heads bobbed. My brother's test results arrived, the jumbled alphabet of a pivotal gene mapped and recorded. I could now report for my own blood draw.

As a nurse at the University of Iowa pulled a needle from my arm and strapped a cotton ball over the tiny puncture, I kept an eye on the vial of blood. It was very pretty; I was amazed by how dark it was. The tube had a pink plastic cap and a pink lovely label, which brought out a deep red behind the blackness. "Go, go, go, you little thing," I whispered.

"What?" asked my genetic counselor, Beverly.

"I was just telling that blood to give me the result I want."

"What is the result you want?" she asked, surprising me. Wasn't it obvious that I wouldn't want to be a carrier? But no choice in reproductive medicine was clear or universal, I was learning. Some people really do want to shape their children right down to height and eye color. Others, like the deaf couple who had been making recent news, wanted a child who would share their condition.

I had been so open-minded when Dan and I first met with

Beverly, comforted by a certainty that any child would be better than no child at all. But somehow, in the six months it had taken to meet up with Luke, get his blood tested, and hear back from the lab, my sense of things had changed. Dan hoped fervently that my DNA would prove mutation-free. Healthy, strong Dan, who sweated so beautifully on a warm day. "Just think how great things could be," he had been saying, "if all this worrying was for nothing." Perhaps because of his sudden, fingers-crossed optimism, my own hopes for good news had leapt skyward.

"Bonnie," Beverly said, cupping her warm hand over my wrist, "you need to think about whether you want to send the bill for this test to your insurance. It's about $350. If you test positive, it might not be in your best interest for insurance companies to know that. You should consider paying out of pocket and keeping the results to yourself." She kept trying to meet my eyes. But I was suddenly so sure my DNA would behave that I told her to go ahead and bill insurance.

Perhaps she sensed that I was in denial. Later we learned that Beverly was somehow moved to wait for my test results before billing.

Several weeks before I had my blood drawn, I did something cavalier. I found myself tempting fate by writing about the moral dilemma Dan and I might face. In my essay I claimed that I was a carrier, as I had always believed I was, even though my testing had not been completed. I grappled with the unpleasant options Dan and I would have to choose among when it came time to start a family. I tried to describe the lessons of my family tree alongside the promises and perils of the genetic testing available to my generation. And I sent the essay off to *The New York Times*, knowing full well that if the HED test came back negative, my essay would have been based on a misconception. But—and this compelled me—if the test returned positive, I would actually experience a little relief in the fact that I hadn't misled anyone, including myself. Somehow, basing the essay on a hypothesis—the diagnosis doctors had given me before genetic testing was possible—allowed me to honestly and thoroughly explore my dilemma. If I had confirmed my carrier status, I realized, I might have been too overwrought to sort through my options rationally and articulately.

When an editor from *The New York Times* called to accept my essay, I was so eager to see my writing appear in the venerable publication that it didn't occur to me to steady myself for the flood of fiery responses my story would provoke. Instead, I set about preparing those around me.

"Is this really okay with you?" I asked Dan, whom the essay portrayed as something of a perfectionist—a man who would prefer to raise robust, athletic children—which was not a true reflection of his sensitivity. Dan gave me a small, proud smile in response. "It's fine," he said. He wanted this as much as I did. He knew our story should be told, and, for a column of fifteen hundred words, he could allow the telling to happen in simplified terms.

Later, I steeled myself for a more difficult phone call. I asked Luke to read the essay—much of which centered on him—and to decide whether I could tell the newspaper to go ahead and publish it. "If you're not comfortable with it, I won't do it," I told him. "You have complete veto power." We hung up so he could read.

As I waited for him to call me back, I reread the piece. I knew it inside out by that point, but I tried to clear my mind and imagine what it would feel like for my brother to read it for the first time.

He would learn that Dan and I had arrived at our options. We could choose to go on in our marriage without children—an option that felt empty to both of us. We could choose to adopt—a trickier prospect. The biological imperative to reproduce spurred us both, though we wanted our babies to be healthy. So, we could spend years saving $25,000 to have my eggs harvested and combined with his sperm. The resulting embryos would be tested for HED, and one or more healthy ones would be placed in my uterus with a 30 to 40 percent chance of implanting—and a chance of twins or triplets. If the expense, anxiety, and physical discomfort of a medical adventure like that seemed too much, we did have another choice, both simple and profound: We could begin a pregnancy in the privacy of our own bedroom. At eleven weeks, via CVS, we could have cells collected from the placenta in order to test our fetus's DNA. A few weeks after that, with test results in hand, we could choose whether or not to continue our pregnancy.

Reading my deliberations about each option, Luke's impression easily could have been that Dan and I wanted to avoid having a child anything like him.

In some ways, we're lucky. HED is no Down syndrome, no cerebral palsy or cystic fibrosis. It doesn't affect mental capacity or motor skills. It doesn't cap life span. The more we talk about HED, the littler it tends to sound. My brother, after all, is healthy and strong, getting good grades in his first year of college. He seems to know the name of every kid he sees on his way to class. In poker, he beats the pants off every guy in his hall and spends his winnings on books and food and, this month, on his first suit; he's taking a smart girl with blond, curly hair to the charity ball.

But Luke grew up in Seattle, where the weather is kind to him nearly all year, where top prosthodontists are plentiful, and where our father has a job with decent dental benefits. Growing up, I came to see HED as a mere inconvenience. Sometimes it brought heavy expenses for our parents, sometimes it caused physical embarrassments for my brother. But it never seemed cataclysmic.

So I fumbled for words recently when I found myself explaining to my brother that Dan and I hope to dodge HED. I wondered if he was thinking, *What's so bad that they'd try so hard to avoid it?*

I breathed shallowly, waiting for the phone to ring and wondering how to keep from resenting Luke for exercising his right to privacy if he asked me not to publish. At the same time, I tried to swallow a lump in my throat as I imagined my baby brother's spirits crumbling with every word he read.

His voice was gravelly when he called back. He was crying.

"I love it," he said.

"What? Why?"

"Because you captured exactly the kind of person I am."

He didn't answer his phone on the Sunday the article appeared, and he returned none of the family's phone calls. I was seeing that my brother did have sorrows about his condition. Surely, he always had. But he kept them to himself, grieving quietly, giving us room to choose oblivion over the hard truth.

With the newspaper in my hands, I reread my essay one more time, thinking of my grandfather. Even though I felt skeptical of afterlife notions, I was still willing to believe that ghosts of the long dead could watch me. What would my grandfather think? In a swift paragraph, I had described his upbringing in the Nebraska heat and his plunge to ruin:

> People considered Earl feeble and tended to him like a baby. He grew into a reckless man, desperate to prove he had no limits— financial, physical, or emotional. He died penniless, addicted to prescription drugs, and alone.

> On our drive home to Iowa from Nebraska, I asked Dan what he thought of what we'd learned.

> "When you think about Earl's life," he said as we whipped through the sweltering summer cornfields, "it seems like we should do whatever we can to avoid passing it on."

E-mails from strangers started popping into my account just hours after the newspaper came out. Scores of mothers and fathers, as well as couples who hoped to become parents, wrote to me from across the country. I read the first messages eagerly, naïvely expecting some kind of reward. But a tone of critical skepticism ran through about half of the letters, and those seized me. Some of the readers grappled with the same questions I posed: Should fate or medicine shape our babies? But most readers believed they knew exactly what Dan and I should do. One called our in vitro option a "no-brainer." Many others, all adoptive parents themselves, called adoption the clear choice for us—implicitly agreeing that HED was best avoided. Other letter writers begged us to forget about testing and allow fate to decide, thereby protecting the gene pool against homogeneity. Many readers really didn't care what we did, as long as we ditched the abortion option. And plenty took issue with the way I compared HED to other disorders.

"As the mother of two children, one of whom has Down syndrome, I found your comments completely offensive," one reader wrote. "I would not trade my son for anything in the world, nor would I change the fact that he has Down syndrome. Your assumptions as to what the quality of life is for people with Down syndrome are ignorant and antiquated."

My stomach began to tighten. Could I handle this?

Several parents of boys with HED also responded with anger, adding to the chorus of voices saying they wouldn't think of trading in their children.

Of course you wouldn't! I wanted to scream. *Goodness knows I wouldn't want you to. But I have a* choice, *you see? If you could have elected for your son to be born with Down syndrome or with HED, would you really have done so?*

I had always known I could embrace the challenges of parenting a child with special needs. It would be, simply, the way life was. Anytime I saw parents with such a child, I knew better than to judge them saintly or downtrodden or anything else. I made no assumptions about whether their family lives were difficult or wonderful or somewhere in between. And while many of these children's health problems were hard surprises for their parents, I knew that plenty of their births were chosen, with all of the information already in hand. I could very well one day be surprised by a birth that would render me the parent of a child with special needs. But with HED, I had choices. It was hard to imagine electing a life of maladies for my child.

I wanted to argue my side, but I'd had my chance. I typed a few heated responses, but never sent them. For a few days, I felt overcome. Responses continued to flow in, all different, all strong, all personal. The only practice I'd had in fielding the commentary of riled readers had been in a few years' experience writing for a little newspaper with a circulation of twenty thousand—nothing like the shelling I was taking now. Still, I was glad I had written the essay before Dan and I had made up our minds about what we would actually do if I turned out to be a carrier. I imagined all the weighing-in I would have invited by revealing an actual decision, as if I were offering it up for judgment and asking for a mass verdict.

With my essay, I had hoped to describe a moral dilemma and give a personal account of how it might look to approach such a problem thoughtfully. But scores of people treated my real-life story as we tend to treat the movies: *She should never have said that. He could have been more courageous. There was too much scenery and not enough sex. It should have been different in the middle. Why couldn't they just sell everything and start over?*

But, I reminded myself, my readers weren't the only ones who approached the essay with a cinemagoer's mentality. The only way I could write it in the first place was to calm myself the way I often did at the movies: by telling myself, *It's not real—I don't have to believe it if I don't want to. At least not yet.*

As I tried to sleep at night, I considered my enormous unknown and crossed my fingers tightly. I begged the universe to surprise me with the unexpected. *May I not be a carrier. May I not be a carrier.*

On a rainy day two months later, I sat down to write Luke's nineteenth-birthday card. After the article had come out, we returned to our usual infrequent but amiable dispatches. The phone rang: a number from the hospital.

"Hi, Bonnie? It's Beverly, your genetic counselor." Something in her voice.

"Hi, Beverly, how are you?" A strange thing in my own sound.

"I wanted to give you good news," she said. Her voice cracked. "But maybe this will be better, so you won't have survivor's guilt. This way, maybe your brother won't be the only black sheep in the family." She took a breath. "The test came back positive. I wanted it to be negative, Bonnie. But you're a carrier."

"Oh, I knew it," I said, trying to sound unfazed. "It seems like I've always known." My favorite thing to do, in fact, was to know things. But over the past year, I had let myself stop knowing. I felt like I had set myself up. I heard Dan, who had been reading under his breath in the next room, fall silent.

"Listen," Beverly said. "You know, this is a wonderful hospital, and now you know your options, so we can help you. You choose whatever is best for you. You and Dan have told us that the cost of in vitro might be out of reach for you. You need to know that no one here will ever judge you if you choose to terminate a pregnancy. We can help you with whatever procedures you choose."

I kept swallowing. No words came.

"I'm sorry," she said.

I walked into Dan's office, where he sat swiveled in his desk chair, facing the door. His face was splotched, his eyes red and wet. My own face burned. Standing before him, I felt shame.

He brought me to his lap, but I couldn't receive any comfort. I sat up straight. Instead of feeling the warmth of his thighs, I felt leg bones on leg bones.

Finally, his voice came through a small space. "What should we do?"

"I don't know," I said. By that point, we felt certain of one thing: We wanted biological children, and we wanted them to be healthy. Our options had boiled down to two: in vitro with preimplantation genetic diagnosis, or a natural pregnancy with the chance of termination.

"I'm so glad we found out now, before we got too desperate for kids," I said, desperate instead to buoy my husband. "We have some time to think."

"Twenty-five thousand dollars for IVF," he said.

"I'm so sorry," I said. But Dan wasn't blaming me or looking back.

"More and more," he said, "I think we should go the other route. It's so much less expensive. We could do it sooner. We could get started."

"That sounds so good on the surface," I said.

"We'd just have to promise ourselves that our plan is our plan," he went on. "We'd have to know ahead of time exactly what we'd do if the test came back positive."

"It sounds so workable, Dan. But when I imagine being pregnant, carrying a child, I'm afraid I'd be unpredictable. I'm afraid I'd fight you. I'm afraid our plan would break my heart."

I pushed myself up from his lap and went to the bathroom. Catching sight of myself in the mirror, I stared. I was different. For the first time, I saw tiny folds of dry skin on my arms and chest. The dark circles under my eyes were not, as a friend had suggested in junior high, a sign that I was "mysterious." They were evidence that I was a carrier. I had always been grateful that the hair on my arms was blond and not too thick. Now, instead of seeing those hairs, I saw their sparseness: the spaces between them. Holding the back of my hand up to the light, I tried to see the signature mosaic pattern in my pores. I tried to imagine how the ridges could be deeper in my fingerprints. *Yes, we are all special,* I thought. *They take great pains to teach us that. But we are not all perfect.* I looked in the mirror, learning myself all over again.

"Defective," I whispered.

This is not a judgment, I thought. *A defect is not a judgment. It is a fact of science, a ripple of biology, with no moral value and no need for defense.* But I didn't believe a word I was thinking.

"Defective," I said again, turning off the bathroom light.

That night, I wrote Luke his birthday card. *And, test results are in,* I added at the end of a mundane note about classes and rain. *I found out today that you and I have part of an X chromosome in common. Thank you for walking with me through this. I would know so little if it weren't for you.*

Some readers of my *New York Times* piece waited weeks, even months, to contact me. Unlike the initial slew of reactions, the last letters were so openhearted and thoughtful that I began writing back. One writer, a college-age woman who suffered from the exceedingly rare female form of ectodermal dysplasia (ED), sent a simple message of gorgeous prose:

> I have ED, and as I start to look ahead in my future, I know that I will be confronted with the same choices that you write about. My mother, my two sisters, and myself are all too familiar with ectodermal dysplasia, knowing the dental bills I racked up, the soccer games I spent on the bench because of overheating, telling people that they shouldn't be jealous that I have no arm hair, and figuring out how to explain my missing front teeth after it was no longer normal for me or my peers to be missing teeth. Our prosthodontist now receives our Christmas cards, graduation party invitations, and praise. I watch TV with closed

captioning and sport hearing aids to counter a 30 percent hearing loss that is a result of ED.

I am a thriving twenty-two-year-old, but every day that I brush my priceless dental implants, I am reminded of the sum total of character-building ED-related challenges that I have dealt with. I am so grateful that my parents were willing to do everything in their power to correct the superficial side effects and to comfort me when I was increasingly aware of what made me a little bit different. I believe that I am a better version of myself because of the small hurdles that I have cleared, but I share your hope that modern medicine can eliminate them for my own children.

Another young woman, a nursing student, reminded me of thoughts I had carried with me as a girl:

I have always had strong feelings toward the topic of genetic selection of embryos simply because I know that I would not have my brother if this was routinely practiced. He is one of the most wonderful people I have ever known, and to think that he would have been disregarded simply for not having sweat glands breaks my heart. My mom likes to tell the story of when I had some basic testing done when I was younger and they told me that I was probably not a carrier. I almost started crying, and my mom asked me what was wrong. I told her that I really wanted to have a baby like my brother. I was quite disappointed to hear that I might not be able to.

As a little girl, I, too, had a quick response for anyone who remarked on Luke's ethereal looks: "I would love to have a baby like him someday." My mother had told me that, yes, I possibly could. And, years later, the test confirmed it: Half of my eggs carried the mutation for the condition. Therefore, statistically speaking, one in four of my pregnancies would produce a healthy girl. One in four would produce a healthy boy. One in four would produce a carrier daughter like myself. And one in four would be a boy with HED.

I was smitten with my brother from the day my parents brought him home from the hospital and centered him on the kitchen table, swaddled to the cheeks, in a blue bouncy chair. He quickly got used to my crushing smooches. Now, nineteen years later, I still stung with affection for him: so smart, funny, tall, fluid, strong. I loved his wildly perfect impressions at our holiday meals and the way he would swoop from his great height to catch the family cat so swiftly, just to snuggle her. He seemed to shrug at any suggestion that a man should hide his heart. My brother, I reflected from our two thousand–mile divide, was real and deep and loving and complex and pained and young and cool-eyed, and his creativity made the very sight of him kaleidoscopic at times. Yes, I would love a son like him. And I had heard other carriers say the same. But, I now wanted to ask them, is the question really about you? Is it really about how much you would like your child? Of course you would adore any child you bear. But have you tried to imagine the pain your son might suffer in order to be the child you're proud to wish for?

What makes a life go wrong? I had begun to wonder. Not genes themselves, but how people react to the ways those genes are expressed. It wasn't a saddle nose, or unusual teeth, or exhausted-looking eyes that made a person shy and full of self-loathing, determined to prove himself. Genes manifested only in flesh and blood. People made them meaningful by judging them good or bad, beautiful or ugly, strong or weak. I knew my future children would be judged by others regardless of whether they had HED, but I felt compelled to block any harm I could.

I was considering preventing the birth of a particular child because of the interpretations others might make upon the sight of his face. In the future of my fears, those interpretations would become a kind of truth for my son—and for the people who were supposed to love him. I knew that if someone told him that he was sick, he would feel sick. If they told him that he was weak, he would feel weak. If they told him that he was ugly, he would search desperately for ways to look handsome. And if he told them that he believed he was handsome already, they might not care.

I promised myself that if I had a son with HED, I would never confess to him my guilt, but I knew he would intuit my unending, silent apology. He would feel me crushing him in a shroud of protection just as he tried to unfurl his fragile wings. He would sense my guilt because I would worry too much about his nutrition. I would obsess too much about the quality of his sleep, and the stylishness of his clothes, and what the children said at the bus stop. (*Have they called you Cancer Boy? Have they said that you look dead?*) I would come too early to pick him up, hovering in the gym doorway to see if the other boys passed him the ball, listening vigilantly to the tones in the girls' voices as they chattered around the drinking fountain, stepping aside so he could soak his T-shirt. In summer I would ply him with spray bottles and fans. In winter I would supply too much lip balm and force him to button his coat against the wick-dry air. One day I might tell him, as if I happened to think of it just then, that he could use my concealer on the shadows beneath his eyes. That he could use my makeup pencils to draw in eyebrows if he ever felt like it. I might be angry when he doesn't moisturize his eczema, instead opting to scratch and bleed at night. I might yell when he doesn't use saline in his nose, even though it would make him sneeze and gag. I would believe that he was choosing to have others not like him. I would busily want all children to adore him at all times. He would know that other children—children without genetic disorders—have sinus and skin problems, too. And he would know that children don't often judge each other for red skin rashes and soft breath smells. He might even try to convince me of this, with a cool wisdom in his eyes, but so immersed in my project of preventing his life from going wrong, I might not hear his wisdom.

In the weeks after my test results came back, I spent more time than ever trying to separate what it might mean to make a decision for my child's sake, and what it might mean to make a decision for my own sake as a parent. But when I was most honest with myself, I found no clear line between those two things. My child's good fortune would nourish me. His sorrows would tunnel my heart. I began to understand that what was tragic could also be best.

Iowa's velvet June evenings reminded us that we had chosen the most difficult time of year to move away. Dan had taken a job in Minneapolis, three hundred miles north, and in just a few weeks, we would be leaving our little Iowa bungalow with its green gardens. I had imagined myself becoming pregnant in the bungalow, wobbling down the spiral staircase to pee every night, laboring in the big claw-foot tub, and eventually changing diapers in the back bedroom. But I had come to realize that if our plans for a family unfolded as we hoped, Minneapolis—a city I had never even visited—would probably become the birthplace of our first child.

As our move approached, I felt a growing dread. I was afraid to leave the bungalow, worried about starting over. Could I get a job quickly enough? Would our new house feel like home? Would the cat run away? As students, Dan and I had enjoyed spending most of our days together, studying, making meals, taking walks. In Minneapolis, with Dan driving across the city to work full-time, how would I see enough of him?

Each time I mounted the porch steps or opened a closet or crossed a room, I felt tugged. This had been our first home together. It had received us in our new marriage, nurtured us with more spirit than I'd ever known a place could hold. We had scrubbed, painted, decorated Christmas trees. We had played string games with our cat on the spiral stairs, chased bats out of the bedroom, rescued baby birds fallen to the garage floor. We had mowed and raked and shoveled. We had stood amazed at overflowing vegetable gardens and planted hundreds of spring bulbs, carrying inside the fruits of our toil: tulips in spring, dahlias in July, cucumbers in August, melons in September, pumpkins in October. We had answered to trick-or-treaters and timed our morning study breaks to coincide with the mailman's halloo. I had baked ovenloads of zucchini bread and chocolate-chip cookies; Dan had trimmed hedges and mulched my hydrangea and sealed out winter's slicing drafts. Certainly all of this came from our love of the house, but more from our love for each other. The gleaming vegetables were mere produce until I shared them with Dan after class. Then they became gifts. And when Dan spent a long afternoon pulling weeds and edging the lawn, the job was only finished when he brought me outside to approve the "national park" he'd groomed for me. The bungalow had been our first physical collaboration, our opus before embarking on parenthood.

On those last June nights, we sat on the deck and watched the fireflies rising high into the evergreen treetops against a cerulean sky. Cicadas trilled. I pined to plant vegetables but instead simply stared at the plot I kept weed bare for the new owner. I deliberated: Would my hydrangea survive such a long transfer? And I mourned: Would anyone tend the Estonian clematis as I had, training it carefully up the porch columns?

Fresh stars pricked the sky, one by one. I now knew I was a carrier of HED. I now knew much more about what the disorder could mean for a child of ours. And even though I could barely picture a life in Minneapolis, I wanted that city to be the place where a child—a healthy child—would make us three.

* * *

I continued to process Earl's story, ironing out details and straining toward his slippery truth. I still called my mother almost every day, prodding her for recollections and coaxing her to flesh out the memories that our family folklore had come to abbreviate.

"Thank you for doing this," she said one afternoon. "This has been a year of great healing for me." I knew that the healing I offered was probably only a salve, but I hungrily accepted her approval. It had been years since we'd spent so much time talking to one another.

I knew my mother wanted me to somehow solve the puzzle of her damaged girlhood, and she still wanted a particular detail: proof that her father had killed Junior. It was a near-satisfying excuse for his failures, because it took the place of the only other explanation she had ever known: that he just didn't love his family. To her, committing murder would be so rattling that even the most dedicated father would struggle to continue in his everyday role. Desperate for a new version of the story, my mother plied me with conspiracy theories. Part of me already saw a less dramatic truth emerging, but another side of me wanted to remain, eyes closed, in the embrace of our frenzied collaboration.

"Your dad has an idea," she said one night. "Junior couldn't handle his jealousy anymore and finally made a move for Esta. Earl was so angry and felt so betrayed that he went wild—he was probably out of his mind with drugs anyway—and he shot Junior."

"Wow, there's a thought," I said.

"You know what my mom told me?" she offered on another occasion. "She always felt something was strange about the female chemist who invented Enz-All. Maybe she had something to do with Junior's murder, right next to all those cans of Enz-All in the warehouse."

"Hmm," I said. "Could be." But I had already come to the

conclusion that the chemist had a bad reputation with Esta and Earl simply because my grandparents were intimidated by such a stark and smart single woman, going it alone in a man's world and succeeding.

Still, I wanted Junior's story to be more glamorous than suicide. At night when my imagination roamed, I pictured all manner of fascinating crime. My mother's family had always claimed there was a mafia conflict in Earl's past. I didn't discount this, knowing that Greeley in its meatpacking heyday was rife with corrupt political alliances and powerful money-lending cahoots. My mom had many times related a clear memory of threatening men arriving at night, pulling black cars into the driveway with their headlights off, which certainly fit my mental image of mob activity. So what would the mob want with my grandfather, or with Enz-All? My wildest idea came as I sat in my office late one night, reading about the chemicals in the product's formula. *Maybe*, I thought, *Enz-All was a compound the mafia wanted because it could dissolve organic matter without leaving a trace.* I remembered stories of mobsters liquefying bodies in oil drums. Or was Earl connected with organized crime in some duller way, as a money launderer? More likely, as Jack suggested, Earl had simply accepted loans from exactly the wrong sorts of people. Yes, maybe my grandfather was late to repay his debts, causing the bad guys to kill Junior as an example—as if to say, *If you don't pay, this'll be your wife and kids.*

I offered these dramatic scenarios to my mother, taking her eager horror as a reward. And even when I accepted that none of these ideas was likely, I tried to believe the relatively simpler conspiracy theory that Junior's family had offered me: "We always figured Earl killed him for the money," his uncle Art had told me. Hardworking people who had come from very little means, Junior's relatives exalted his success at Dow Chemical.

"He had money. A lot of money," Art said.

"Now where did that money go?" asked Art's wife, Alice,

raising an eyebrow. "There was nothing left for any of us. Doesn't that almost prove it?"

I wanted them to be right. I wanted the story to be full of intrigue, full of backstabbing and low, dark dealings. Somehow, I felt that a sinister family history could give me something outside of myself on which to pin my reproductive decisions. But it was becoming more and more clear that the less dramatic versions of Earl's story were the more likely. Phone conversations with my mother were no longer reinforcing and sometimes grew tense.

"You do have to realize, it really was strange," she pressed. "It was as if my dad really forgot about Junior after we left Greeley, except for these glimmers every few years that really tortured him. Doesn't that mean anything to you?"

It did—perhaps too much. I knew that if I wanted plain answers, I needed to try something different. One afternoon, I decided to call Betsy, the ex-wife of Earl's friend Calhoun, who had died in 1995. She still lived in the Cheyenne house where Junior had clamored against the front door, desperate for a fix when his usual supplier—my grandfather—was incapacitated by his own drug habit.

Just moments into the phone call, I was struck by Betsy's lucidity compared with my grandmother's patchy recollections. While my grandmother had no trouble talking in detail about family buzz and current events, her memories of a painful past were so hazy that I had almost been fooled into believing it was just too hard for anyone to remember what life had been like forty years earlier. But Betsy's memories were unmuddied by ideas of what she should or shouldn't have seen or heard or done. She simply told me what she remembered.

"I think it was a suicide," she said of Junior's death. "He was very depressed. I know quite a bit about depression, and I can tell you that Junior just did not see the future. I had shock treatments for my own depression. Supposedly, shock treatment makes you forget the bad things. And for me, it saved my life. I would not be alive now if I hadn't gone through that, because the depression was reaching a suicidal level. I had just gotten out of the hospital when Junior died. Calhoun didn't want me to go up and look in the casket. He was afraid it would send me back."

I asked her to tell me more.

"Junior was very smart," she continued, "and he had such a good job with Dow Chemical. But I'm pretty sure he lost the job because he was acting really abnormal. Paranoid. He just couldn't work. His coworkers were scared of him. They had to let him go. When he died, it hit Earl and Calhoun hard. They felt they should have seen the signs. It just spiraled downhill; maybe Junior and Earl were spiraling together. I wish I had been more observant."

Betsy's clear, simple honesty made me crave more. "What else do you remember about that time?"

"I keep thinking . . . I remember so well when your grandparents and your little mom lived in Greeley in that big, big, big house by the lake. I was so envious. Let me tell you, we were struggling so much. To me it looked like the biggest house I'd ever been in. They had us over for dinner, and the kids would play so nice together. Then later they moved up here to Cheyenne, into an old broken-down thing. We visited them, and everyone was ill at ease. We were doing so much better, and they had gone the other way. I remember Earl would leave all of us and go down into the basement. I suppose that was for the drugs."

"What do you remember about my grandfather?"

"You do know about his congenital problems? No teeth, no body hair, no sweat glands . . . which can't help but form your mind, your personality, everything. And he had a superior intellect. It just makes a bad combination. Because of his physical strain, he couldn't do everything his brain wanted him to do. He and Junior were two of a kind that way. It had to be terribly frustrating. Your grandfather had so many ideas. I think Calhoun

and I put $500 into the Nebulizer—it was all we could afford—
and then it didn't go anywhere. The money we lost would have
been two or three thousand dollars nowadays. I thought we were
going to get rich. And we all probably should have; I don't know
why it didn't happen. I just know that your grandfather wanted
to get involved in everything and anything, if it meant he was
accepted socially. Don't you think growing up with all of his
medical conditions did a number on his self-esteem? Think of
what that would do to a boy."

Betsy's memories of 1962 were like water, unremarkably following the path of least resistance. *The truth usually is that way,*
I thought after we hung up. We marvel when life is stranger
than fiction because we're accustomed to a reality that is most
often predictable and most often makes logical sense. Life is not
a carefully crafted narrative, built like a romance novel or mystery show. It is a flow of experience in which each character simply tries to survive. Most often, in whatever plotting people do,
they aim for life stories of tranquility and satisfaction—not tales
of high drama and dark twists.

Outside of the quiet observations I had shared with Dan,
Betsy might have been the first person to bluntly propose that
a man's physical condition could lead directly to his personal
failures. Hearing her baldly state the idea that I had barely dared
suggest made me feel I was finally getting somewhere.

I had recently found the words *a man shot* at the center of a
page of Earl's notes. In the last years of his life, my grandfather
was clearly still haunted by a memory emblazoned, then crudely
scratched away, of his dead friend.

"Your dad," I carefully tried to explain to my mother, "blamed
himself for Junior's death."

"But did he kill him? Did my dad kill him?"

The more I had learned about Junior, the more it seemed that
he would have been diagnosed with schizophrenia today. Several
people I interviewed remembered his strange paranoia in his last

weeks as a Dow employee—just before he went to work with my grandfather. For the sake of my story, and for my mother's peculiar path to peace of mind, I wanted Junior's complaints to have been true: that his bosses and coworkers were watching him, threatening him, and toying with his loyalty by giving him top-secret projects that led the government to monitor him. I wanted to believe that Junior and my grandfather were scientists with complicated, specific secrets that I could discover—not simply two young men wracked physically and mentally by the pressures of their jobs, the strain of disease, and the angst of addiction. The drugs my grandfather gave Junior might have eased his mental illness, or might have hurt, and perhaps did both. "But," I finally mustered the courage to tell my mother, "it makes clinical sense that Junior would have felt suicidal at times."

"No," she said, refusing to let me close the case that, left open, was a lifeline for her. "I think we should hire a psychic. There's got to be more to this story."

I tried to reassure her that her new compassion for her father could remain. Despite making mistakes that shook him to the core, he loved his family and wanted the same storybook life that his wife and children yearned for. Earl's spirit was crippled by Junior's death because he blamed himself for driving his friend to ruin. Desperate to prove himself, he had taken Junior's personal resources—his money, his trust, and the last of his health. Even if he didn't pull the trigger that April night, my grandfather felt as if he had.

On one of our last evenings in Iowa, watching the lightning bugs flickering to life on the lawn, I brought Dan up to date on Earl's life as I was coming to understand it.

"What do you think about all that?" I asked him. "I mean, when you think about us having kids?" My pulse always quickened when I asked him a difficult question, because I knew he wouldn't sugarcoat the answer.

"Well," he said, "I think no matter what story you believe, it's pretty clear that a kid with this condition doesn't get a good start in life."

It seemed so sensible when he said it. In a strange way, Dan's words felt like permission of some kind for me. Family loyalty had me continually reminding myself that my grandfather and my brother were real, distinct people—unique individuals, not poster boys for life with HED. I had long refused to believe that my grandfather's struggles could reappear in my brother's life. So why would I entertain the possibility that they could repeat for my children? For all my roaming, I hadn't fallen far from the tree after all. Just like my mother, I had things I wanted to believe and things I didn't. Dan, however, saw our risk plainly.

earl

They took me to Denver, to Mount Airy, a psychiatric hospital.
Sick in a way, the clarity that comes, I thought to myself,
lying in my crisp white bed as I waited to meet the doctor. *I had
a simple question, preceded by simple facts: Junior was my best
friend. Esta was my wife. Paula, Greg, and Curt were my children. Junior had no wife, and no children. Does merit build this
way? Does forgiveness fall accordingly?*

The day before, the deputy had said, "That's all we have for
now, Mr. Hickman. We know where to find you if we have more
questions. Now do you have any questions for us?"

Junior's blood stained the floor at our feet.

"No, thank you, sirs," I had answered, standing in the doorway. "Best of luck with the investigation. Looks simple as suicide
to me, but I'm no expert."

But what I really wanted to ask was, "How does merit build?"

I looked around me in the hospital room, at the wires and
the square-tiled wall and the leaves on the other side of a thick
windowpane. When Montgomery had come to the house earlier
that day, I thought he was bringing good wishes. I thought he

would come inside and shake my hand and say, "Listen, man, I can't imagine what it would be like, getting questioned in the death of my own best friend."

He did shake my hand, but his words went past me, to my wife. "Esta, Earl needs a rest," he said. "Helman and I, we're going to take him for a rest."

I had a flash of deer in the mountains. I exhaled, happy.

But now I knew why he spoke only to Esta, and why he pressed my back with his hand as we went down the walk, and why Esta pushed the door shut with her phony cheer bouncing all over Mrs. Montgomery.

That night, when the staff explained the electroshock process, I still believed they would treat me like a man. I thought I had a say.

"Look, sirs, not to be ungrateful," I told them, "but I've got a best friend getting buried on Saturday. I'm to be a pallbearer, so I must attend."

"That's all right," one of the doctors said, not looking at me, just straightening the pages in my file. "Don't you worry about it."

Then he gave the sort of smile that's for children, when you promise them one thing before doing another.

I had to sign long documents, and then they could give me capsules to relax the muscles. I was to sign the documents before each treatment. It would be approximately three weeks, they said, before signs of improvement could be ascertained.

The food there was nice. I remember that. But before each treatment, I could not eat for twelve hours. "I suppose I can eat in the morning, before the funeral?" I asked on the first Friday. The nurse just nodded, absent.

I was a man familiar with medicine, and therefore I fretted and carped less than the average patient. They might have appreciated me more. Seconal was a drug I knew, and electroconvulsive therapy had principles I understood. I knew it could be difficult, but I also knew it could create peace. If that treatment was the thing that could help me rest, make my addiction end, allow me to return to that moment when the sky was pink and my wife sang at the sink with our children buzzing around the blue television glow—just those things—then yes. I signed agreeably each time, thinking of them, my family. I signed and signed. I signed anything they put in front of me.

Helman came every few days. They let him watch. The intern brought me capsules to swallow. "Take out your dentures, Mr. Hickman," he always ordered. I felt so red-hot in the cheeks each time, even before we began. All the machines in such a small room, each one a little furnace alive and zizzing.

The windows were all sealed tight, and I wasn't sure if they could open at all, but as I never received an answer, I asked each time they prepared me, attaching the electrodes. "It's awfully hot," I would say. "I don't sweat, see."

"Right, Mr. Hickman," the intern would say. "Let's have those teeth now. Good."

My eyes would follow as he dropped them on the tray, never putting them in water.

Dr. Ebaugh appeared for my time on the machines. "This should be nothing, Earl. You should do just fine, all right? Any questions?"

He was so relaxed and certain, so sturdy and glowing gold and far away.

"Awful hot," I told him.

"All right, well, this'll be over in no time. You just relax. Easier with the Seconal, isn't it? Wise of you to take it. We get patients who refuse, and they end up broken-boned and toothless, poor fools. Now this over the temples is graphite-conductive salve, and these are just small electrodes inside the patches. Nice and easy. And there you are, wise again as you close your eyes. See you shortly," he'd say.

The first time, it was a grass fire.

And then we were back. "Quite a roomful of equipment, you gentlemen," I smiled. So they would know my mind was clear and strong. They asked me questions right away.

"Clever," I said, "but yes, sirs, I believe I do know who I am. Give me just a moment, and I will tell you. First: I was a grass fire and the barn burned and the house burned and my mother burned in the house. No, I do not recall her name. I'm not certain it was my mother, but I know it was my grass fire, and quite a bit of smoke. Terribly too warm."

A good sleep was all I needed. By the time I awoke, Junior was in the ground.

I told Ebaugh the next time, "Of course I'd be happy to sign. You are a good man, Doctor, that I do not doubt. But you do understand that I don't like to be where it's so hot? You understand I don't sweat? It's a condition I was born with. Yes, I will sign every time. Why wouldn't I?"

He said he thought I was improving already. He said he thought the basketball was lost in the wheat and was burst in the wheat and lay like smashed beetle wings. And with their beaks the hens pecked one of their own, all the way to a bloody pulp. I remember my throat saying *kah*, and they finally put a wet rag on my neck though I told them no, no, by now I need a river.

"Good to meet you," I said to my visitors. I didn't know anything for certain.

"That's funny," I said. "I never forget a face. Anyway, how can I help, officers?"

They said I had reported the previous week that a man named Junior was despondent and told me he felt like going out and shooting himself. "Well, if I said it, I said it," I answered. But I certainly couldn't think of a man named Junior that day. Except my old friend, but he was gone, and no one knew what had happened to him. They asked me to certify that I was indeed Earl Lee Hickman, born in Nebraska.

It wasn't the fire in my head. It wasn't the muscles hard as mahogany. It wasn't the ulcers from wearing dry dentures. It was the burning on my face and in my chest, so terribly hot.

"Can you cool it somehow?" I asked the nurses, finally feeling afraid. "With ice on my neck perhaps? You don't suppose there's a way to help the lip cracking either? A jelly or ointment, for example?"

They would say anything, as long as I signed.

Whh. Whh. Sssah. The top of a creek, the sun as the water: jumping to catch the bright and diving to catch the shadow. Strobing, peculiar, the image of a beer can under the surface. I reached in with my arm not attached to the rest of my arm, and I had to feel around for the can because it wasn't where it seemed, flashing there in the creek, and blessed heaven: Up came the can and out poured cold black mud.

By the second week, when he came in, I said, "Good to meet you, Mr. Helman. Oh, *Dr.* Helman. An honor."

And, "Property? I don't have any property. That's for certain."

And, "Well then, I suppose it's as you say. I've nothing to lose. What shall I sign these by?"

And he told me how my signature reads: *Earl L. Hickman.*

"You hold on to these autographs now," I told Helman and the others standing by. "They'll be worth millions someday. Perhaps you didn't know you're looking at the inventor of the Adjustable Foot Rest for Polio Bed Patients. It's patented. No, I am not pulling your leg."

I bantered because I was embarrassed. My signature was nowhere in my hand. I couldn't remember its shape. But I marked each page. I tried to cooperate. I did just as they asked. They plainly found me childish. I was abashed for them. With tact, with jokes, I tried to help them save face. To remind them that we were equals.

One of the afternoons, *thwuh, pat,* the sound of a rock sailing from my slingshot onto the bull's white flank. The bull huffed and trotted a heavy thump to the corral gate, and my father said, "What are you thinkin', kid? Where's your mother?" Well, what I was thinkin' was, *Least he could say "nice shot,"* seeing the bull stood so far back in the pen.

Oh she was lovely, with red lips, and she was gentle, and her hands were cool. She said Esta, Esta. It's Esta. All I needed was to be reminded. My beautiful wife. She said the next time she'd bring the children. Children! She said, "Earl, you look so good and pink-cheeked, and you're filling out. What a nice white uniform they have you in. Like when you drove the ambulances. Remember?"

This would become her work. Reminding me, event by event, of my life. Choosing carefully her omissions.

The kids came with Esta the time after that. Paula brought me a picture. She said, "Mom told us you need help remembering. This is the house. These are the ducks. And remember little Curt?"

When I saw Greg, I shook his hand and I said, "You say you are *my* son? Not possible!"

Esta told me he cried. I scared him when I said he couldn't possibly be mine. He thought I had forgotten him. But I only meant he was so good-looking and strong, it was hard to believe he came from me.

The doctor finally said, "Six weeks, nine treatments—you're a textbook case, Earl, open and shut, healthy as a horse."

I did feel awfully good. When I got home from the hospital, I loved myself in the mirror. I filled my clothes a little more. I was better than just the color of an old typewriter page.

I told Esta we should go ahead and see if Joyce and Jim wanted to come up from Broomfield with the boys that Saturday. "We can visit all afternoon and have dinner and play cards," I said, watching surprise grow in her eyes, even a little suspicion.

"The kids can play," I said. "I'll stay home with you the rest of this week. You're my sweetheart. Worn out from these kids all the time, aren't you? We'll have Joyce and Jim on Saturday, and I'll wait all the way to Monday before I start doing any work again."

It must have been the last time she felt happy I was off work. It was for me, too.

Joyce and Jim had good amazed looks on their faces when they saw me. Esta took the awkwardness away, just saying it plain: "Doesn't Earl look fine? Fat and healthy!"

"What's for dinner?" I said in the middle of lunch, and they all laughed.

That afternoon I said, "Joyce, Jim, why don't I take you for a drive? We can go see all the Hickman business holdings around Greeley. Would you like to see that?"

We got in the car, and something told me to just skip stopping by the warehouse to show off the Enz-All, even though I had been told all was well in there, and the stacked cans and their labels were still clean and bright. Of course they were. What could have soiled them?

We started at the bowling alley instead. Odd—we all laughed with confusion—my key wasn't going in. Sticky lock. "Anyway," I told them, "this is Classic Lanes. We can come back in a few hours when it opens, if you like. We can bowl a game on the house."

We piled back into the car and drove over to 2020, the medical building. It was of course locked up for the weekend. But this was when I felt a thud in my stomach. My key didn't work there, either. I could see a shine; the slot was new.

"This is very strange," I told Joyce and Jim. I could hear my voice trembling. I know they heard it, too. I knew better than to go on. I should have taken them back to the house right then.

Jim said, "We don't have to do this now, you know, Earl."

But I had to know. The pharmacy and the motel and the service station and the two little rental houses. My keychain swung in the ignition, heavy and worthless.

* * *

The lawyer said, "That's preposterous, really. They can't do that. I'll see about this right away."

"Thank you," Esta said, the pinch in her voice finally loosening.

A week later, the lawyer said, "Sit down please, Mr. Hickman, Mrs. Hickman." He pulled up a second chair for my wife. "I'm very sorry," he said. "There's nothing to be done. All of the property is gone. Look. You signed it over, Mr. Hickman. Is this not your signature? You signed here, and here, and here."

The worst part was Esta's voice, slowly disappearing. "The house?" she whispered that night, the curtains blowing as if this were any other night in any other year.

"You and the kids will be all right," I whispered back. "You're to sign a homestead deed. Then the bank can come after me but not after you. I think."

Her whispers were more like scrapes. Her throat sounded rotten. "The loans?"

"Pay it all back," I said. "I'll have to. Every penny."

"I'll have to go back to work," she said.

"No," I said. "Not yet." I would come up with something. Some way to recover everything and give them even more.

A few days later, Paula was sitting on the porch, watching bees or doing whatever she liked to do out there while she stared into the garden in the sun. I watched her before she saw me. She talked to herself. She seemed happy, in her own world. I wanted to scoop her into my arms, eat all that joy. I didn't realize she would hate so much to be interrupted. I had a handful of the plastic dial-a-pack dispensers we planned to sell with the Enz-All tablets. I owed too much on the Enz-All endeavor. It was over. But how could I use my inventory?

"Paula?" I said.

I held out a dial-a-pack. She and Greg had helped me snap together so many hundreds of them in the warehouse. "What is this?" I asked.

"What?" she said, jerked from her fantasy.

I pushed the gadget into her hands. "Can you think of any-thing this could be used for?"

She looked at me.

"Like a toy or a game or something?"

"No," she said.

At my desk, my pencil was empty, the pages were blank, my files were thin. All of my beginnings were dead. There was no time for a new start.

"Get a job," Esta said. "Anything."

"It's too much," I said. "We owe too many people. Not all the best people."

"I don't want to hear this," she said.

"Any more than I want to say it."

"What are you going to do?"

"Something," I said. "I don't know. I just can't think. I just need something to help me think."

"Oh my God, Earl," she said. "Not again. Give those to me. Don't let the kids see you sleeping when the sun is up." But already I saw beyond her pleading eyes, to a place outside the pressure. She wailed when she saw me crawling to the couch.

"Esta, shh," I said that night before bed. She was as stiff and cold as I had ever felt her. "Just please. Push your fingers over my neck, please. I'm sorry. Please."

Each daybreak, I knew there was one proper thing I could do: have breakfast with my family before Paula and Greg went to school. It was so hard. I had to imagine the kids' noisy voices as marionette strings to my limbs. For them, I would leap to life and dance.

But some days it was almost impossible to rise to the swarms of mail and clattering phone and plague of door chimes. I had to tell the kids. I had to say it somehow, but I didn't want to scare them, little blond things. But what if I said nothing, and it hap-pened that day?

So I pulled my rubbing bones to the table and sat. And I said, "All right, Paula, Greg, can you listen to me for a minute?"

I saw Esta look over, and I had the strange feeling she knew what I would say.

"Listen, you kids. When you walk to school, walk straight there. And in the afternoon, walk straight home. Don't dilly-dally. Don't stop in the park. Always walk with your friends and don't go alone. Never talk to strangers. Never get in anyone else's car. Do you understand? You have to be very, very careful."

"Of what?" Paula asked.

"Of kidnappers," I said. "Esta, you, too."

Into my wife's face flooded a low gray dread that I had never seen before.

In Minneapolis we would learn to use sidewalks. Our street wasn't busy, but it wasn't quiet either. For the first few months in our new home, I ached for the Iowa bungalow. I dreamed I knocked on the door and no one answered. I dreamed I went unwelcome to parties hosted by strangers there. I dreamed of the yard and my flowers and the view from our honey-lit bedroom. We had been hard-pressed to find fault with our first home, but our new house offered plenty to make us wonder whether we'd made a mistake. The mortgage was almost three times as high for a house that was only a smidgen larger. Though flush with established perennials, the yard was too small and shady for a vegetable garden. Funky wallpapers needed to come down; basement mold needed killing; the crumbling driveway needed replacing; the one-car garage shrugged to one side; and a nerve-wracking, leaky bulge in the living room ceiling hung darkly over our heads and gave the upstairs bedroom a sled-worthy slope.

A week after we moved in, we celebrated my twenty-seventh birthday with burgers and a bottle of wine in the backyard. I still dreamed of becoming pregnant at twenty-eight; Dan was two months shy of turning thirty, the age at which he had always imagined starting a family. We felt we had about a year to fall in love with our new home and see it as the perfect place for a baby. And, of course, something like a year to figure out what to do about the HED in my genes.

As we gathered our dishes, a little voice piped from the other side of the fence, "What are you doing?"

I turned to see a round-faced three-year-old with shining, dark hair. His German accent came through as he continued: "I can come to your *haus*?"

His seven-year-old sister helped him cross the flower beds into our yard.

"Do you know what this is?" she asked, pointing to a spiny plant growing from a corner of the garage.

"A weed," I said, already overwhelmed.

"No! It's a raspberry! I promise! You should let it grow for a while and see what happens."

Something began to relax in me. "Okay," I said. "Thanks."

Leo and Delia were my first friends in Minnesota. They visited every day, helping with the garden, baking with me, and bringing artwork to adorn the blank refrigerator.

Later in July, when Dan started work, my sister flew in from Seattle for a long visit. I needed her company as I continued to unpack boxes, and I wanted a companion as I explored my new neighborhood. I was terrified of feeling alone in this new city, and I had been spilling my worries to Amanda over the phone.

When she walked into the house for the first time, she shot me a confused look. "Bonnie, it's beautiful! What's the problem? This is going to be perfect." She set to work arranging my life down to the minutiae. While I arrayed houseplants and decided which pictures belonged on which walls, she patiently pieced together my long-overdue wedding album. And on the second morning, she told me it was time to start walking the lake.

Four blocks from our new house lapped the southwestern corner of Lake Harriet, which would become the anchor of my life in Minnesota. Amanda walked with me before I had a routine, before I fell into the habit of traveling counterclockwise, before I learned to recognize faces of my fellow lake walkers and their myriad dogs. And while I panted through the heavy, wet summer heat on my way to regaining a fitness I hadn't known in years, my sister might have been the first to point out all the strollers. "This is Kid Central," she said, loping alongside me. "You're going to love it."

Slowly, week by week, I began to see what she saw, all within walking distance of our house: dozens of young moms circling the lake with jogging strollers; neighborhood playgrounds just blocks apart, each with kid-crammed wading pools sparkling blue; a busy beach full of three-foot-tall sandcastle builders and their chatting parents; two ice-cream shops; three toy stores; a bookstore just for children, complete with cats and chickens roaming between the shelves; nightly summer concerts at the lake's edge; shore spots perfect for duckling spotting and bobber plopping; even a six-inch-high door in the base of a tree trunk on the path, whose elfin resident responded to hundreds of letters a year from folks in the neighborhood. All you had to do was put your letter inside the door, and a few days later your response would be among scores inside, typed on matchbook-size paper. I thought of writing to the elf to ask for advice on how to let go of the bungalow I missed so much. But as soon as I had that thought, something shifted.

By the time my sister returned to Seattle two weeks later, walking around Lake Harriet had become my habit. One morning, I realized I had returned to my front door without checking a single street sign. That day, I pushed my beautiful antique library table into place beneath the sunny window in my writing room. For a moment, I worried that too many months in the sunlight would fade the wood. But then I heard myself think, *We'll be putting the crib here pretty soon anyway.*

Soon after, weeding my way through the backyard, I found that Delia's vine bore a single ripe raspberry. The same day, we had our broken dishwasher replaced. When I opened the door and saw the new utensil basket with its hinged plastic topper, I surprised myself by imagining baby-bottle parts snapped securely inside.

At that moment, I realized that somewhere between Lake Harriet, weedy flower beds, and a pileup of dirty dishes, I had stopped picturing the bungalow when I thought of home. It was time to prepare for family.

As winter came on, I called the doctor's office to arrange a checkup, asking the receptionist to schedule me with a practitioner she considered warm. "I have some genetic concerns I'm sensitive about," I explained. "I just want to see someone who's a good listener and who can help me talk through my situation a little." Talking to a doctor about getting pregnant felt like a first step. I wanted to start telling my story, but only in circumstances that felt protected and confidential. I was looking for wisdom in earnest now.

Later that week, I waited in the exam room. I couldn't help but smile when the doctor entered the room. She was short and slight, with a tumble of hair the color of crane fly wings. Her nametag was pinned upside down.

"Hi there," Dr. Kelson said, extending her hand.

Within moments, I was busy describing HED, which was unfamiliar to most doctors I met. She seemed struck by the fact that Dan and I had already done so much legwork: learning what the disorder is like, finding out my carrier status, teasing out our options. She did indeed seem warm, and I decided to ask her advice. Now, whenever I found a person I trusted to be thoughtful, I burned to ask, "What would you do?"

I laid out our dilemma, then circled back to the beginning. "First of all," I said, "I can't stand the message this choice seems to send about my brother and my grandfather, as if their lives aren't valuable. Their lives are precious to me."

"But this is not your grandfather or your brother you're choosing against," she said.

A whole new person, then. A new person about whom I could only cherry-pick clues from the lives of those who had been like him, in perhaps only a single way. Once again, I faced the problem of choosing the right prophecy. My son could be an inventor with an excruciatingly tender soul, like my grandfather. He could be a quick-witted jokester with miles of perception, like my brother. He could be a loyal, trusting spirit with a catching laugh, like Dan.

Then I flashed on my grandfather in the psychiatric hospital, trapped, his wondrous mind burned by electrodes again and again. I thought of my little brother, too hot to cry as a baby in his first summer. I remembered him standing at the school bus stop, stoic and small, to begin receiving the education that his enormous mind swallowed easily—along with barbs from his schoolmates.

Sitting in Dr. Kelson's office, I was reminded of Dan's words as we considered Earl. "I'm sure our son would never see the inside of a mental institution simply because of his disorder," he said. "But maybe we should just ask ourselves what would be most loving. I think the most loving thing we could do is give our kids the best shot at a good life from the very beginning."

Dr. Kelson listened as I talked my way back and forth between a natural pregnancy with the chance of abortion—our inexpensive, almost unfathomable option—and preimplantation genetic diagnosis—our terribly costly option with no guarantees. I knew the doctor could see the way I squirmed every time I said the word *abortion*.

"There are some parents," she said, "who, no matter what horrible problem their fetus is diagnosed with, simply would not have an abortion. They say they wouldn't be able to live with themselves."

She left me a moment to think about this, and slowly I got the message. Which would I rather live with: the fact that I had an abortion, or the fact that I knowingly brought into the world a child who would suffer because of his inherited condition? What if I put the pain of these two things side by side? I was surprised to realize that if I were to choose against abortion, it would be for my own sake. Accepting any pregnancy, no matter what, would spare me from the guilt of abortion, and, it seemed, from the judgment of others. As paradoxical as it seemed, choosing against the birth of an affected baby could be a choice for my child's sake; the healthy child who might later be born in his place would never know the pain of HED. Either choice brought with it a terrible weight—in one case the burden would be entirely mine, and in the other, mostly my child's.

Dr. Kelson was generous. Most doctors, I knew, wouldn't have entertained my question, worrying too much about their influence. But she gently helped me to see things from a slightly different angle. Her words were sensitive and carefully chosen, yet I heard a simple and reassuring message: *Why not go the economical, natural route, then terminate a pregnancy if it's not right?* She had heard me say that a baby could be years away if we decided to save up for in vitro and preimplantation genetic diagnosis. And she assured me that while our natural route to a healthy baby would be in many ways agonizing, the medical route could be just as fraught with logistics and anxious hopes.

"But if we went ahead and got pregnant on our own," I told the doctor, "I'm afraid I'd go back on our plan. I'm afraid I wouldn't recognize myself. That I'd be crazy and fierce with motherhood. That I'd fight my husband. That once a child was growing inside of me, I'd say no abortion, no matter what."

She waited while I wiped my eyes and blew my nose. And then she said, "Write it down. Before you become pregnant, make your agreement with your husband. Then put it on paper."

Dr. Kelson was a general practitioner. I would go on to see specialists, so I would not see her again. But her advice was the perfect, gentle wind to keep me sailing until I found my way.

* * *

As I rode the bus to meet Dan for dinner, I was surprised by the lightness I felt. The possibility of conceiving naturally made children seem so much closer. Perhaps pregnancy was only a few months away.

I already felt weakened by the social shame that an abortion might bring, but I felt a tiny giddiness inside as I began to imagine: *Our child. Our son. Our daughter.* And yet, sitting beside those feelings, the possibility of in vitro remained all too comforting to me. Why was I so sure that a medicalized conception would be a good swap for the torment of a wait-and-see pregnancy? And why did in vitro seem like a panacea for the most troubling parts of our dilemma? Because, I suddenly realized, I wouldn't have to feel totally responsible for my choice. Having created embryos by hand from our egg and sperm, doctors— not us—would do the choosing and the discarding in a world so minute that we wouldn't see any carnage.

We also would not be shamed for our choice. While we would feel the need to keep an abortion to ourselves, perhaps we would be able to talk openly about our in vitro experience. The medical option seemed the perfect end run around our moral dilemma. Because embryos are tiny cell blobs, as small as sand and unrecognizable as human, the in vitro process seemed, despite its discomforts and complexities, like the easy option.

So, at dinner, I pressed Dan once again. "Could you explain one more time? Why do you think it seems best for us to go the natural route?" It was warm inside the barbecue shack. The restaurant glowed red, illuminating the churning snowfall outside.

"Here's how I see it," Dan said. "Either we spend months going in and out of clinics, shelling out for a barely better than slim chance of getting pregnant, or we stay at home and do it ourselves, with a 75 percent chance of making a healthy baby."

Dan knew I needed to talk myself through a block. After

answering my question, he just listened, slowly working his way through a pile of spicy ribs and corn bread.

"Not to mention the chance of twins or triplets," I said, continuing Dan's thought about the challenges of in vitro fertilization. "And I know that's not a fun way to get pregnant." I had heard enough stories from friends who had endured fertility treatments to know that the process wasn't painless or quick. Months or even years of drugs, poking, and prodding might lead to a healthy baby, but often they led to another round of treatments—or even defeat. If we were fertile as we assumed, it did seem strange to opt for complicated, uncomfortable treatments just for the ethical advantage I perceived.

"Plus," I went on, "if it doesn't work, we'll lose thousands of dollars and end up trying in our own bed anyway. And then there's always the chance that we'll start by trying in our own bed and end up in the fertility clinic later if we have trouble getting pregnant. But I swear, if we only had the money, it still seems like the perfect thing." I paused and looked at Dan, who wore a peaceful expression as he chewed.

"What if someone handed us $25,000 right now?" I asked. "What would we do with it?"

"Finally fix the bathroom up," he suggested.

"And get that bulge out of the living room ceiling," I added. "Straighten out the whole tilting house."

We both knew we couldn't even accomplish that much with $25,000. Maybe we'd get a second car, use the money to pay back a third of my college debt, or start a college fund for our hypothetical kid. But what we weren't saying, it didn't take long to realize, was "buy a 30 to 40 percent chance at a healthy baby."

I thought this over as I ate my baked beans. "Okay," I said, "but what if we were millionaires? Then what would you want to do about having kids?"

"The same," he said without hesitating. Slowly, I was beginning to see.

I thought of the times I had explained our quandary to doctors, nurses, and close friends, then finished by saying, "It's just a matter of saving a ton of money." For the first time, I saw how I had been using that line to avoid dealing with our difficult alternatives.

As we finished our meal, it dawned on me that something felt cleaner, perhaps more honest, about a plan to achieve a natural pregnancy with the chance that it might come to an early end. Dan was quiet as I finished eating. My thoughts widened. Conception, birth, loss, and death were human experiences people faced every day, without necessarily knowing the right course. The beginnings and endings of lives—perhaps especially lives ended in their beginnings—were trials to meet on one's own terms, carrying one's own story.

I didn't feel ready to write down an agreement, but it felt like Dan and I had come closer to a decision. As we walked out to the car, snow squeaked beneath our shoes.

"Well," Dan said, "if we really are going to try to get pregnant next fall, we need to travel our butts off, starting right now."

His words made me giddy. *Pregnant. Next fall.*

"Sounds great," I said, only faintly realizing that his excitement was for a fresh round of travel—not so much, just yet, the possibility of a baby.

Since we had moved to Minneapolis, Dan had fallen in love with his airline job not least because of the free flying we could do. In his first six months with the company, we had doubled the number of stamps in our passports. In some ways, Dan seemed to be living the footloose life he had always imagined for his twenties. Now, entering his thirties, he felt he was getting the best of all worlds: marriage, a good home in a friendly neighborhood, a decent job, and the freedom to travel almost anytime, anywhere.

"So, where do you want to go this weekend?" he asked.

"Bruges?"

"Sounds good," he said. "I think we're going to have to travel all over when you're pregnant, too."

"We'll see."

As we buckled up, I had a harrowing thought. I saw an image of our little embryo-turning-fetus traveling the world inside of me for three months. If test results returned positive for HED, I imagined myself writing him a letter to say goodbye. Telling our unborn son what he had experienced in his short time with us, I would describe for him a tiny, beautiful existence. Writing that letter would be my penance, my prayer.

Six months later, in June 2006, Dan and I settled into yet another pair of airplane seats, swept up in the whirlwind of travel we had promised each other. In recent weeks, we had visited Los Angeles, Honolulu, Budapest, and our families in Seattle. The following week, we planned a week of camping in Alaska. For now, we were flying to Lake George in upstate New York to spend a weekend sunning, water-skiing, and barbecuing with Dan's extended family.

One reason for the Lake George celebration was the eightieth birthday of Dan's great-aunt, a family matriarch. To honor her, there would be a huge catered dinner on the last night at the lake. As we flew, for the first time I simply wished I was pregnant— without qualification, without reservation. Even though Dan and I had not yet decided to start trying, I wanted, in a mute, old-fashioned way, to show that I was contributing to the family.

I had begun to believe, however, that my first pregnancy would end early. One reason for my pessimism was that I often caught myself thinking that my life was too good. I enjoyed a best friend in my husband, a house of my own, and even the luxury of time to read, write, and walk the lake. Sometimes I wondered when the car crash was going to happen. Saying good-bye to my first pregnancy was the tragedy I kept begging my stray gods to hold at bay.

Because Dan and I always hoped to have more than one child, I expected to have more than one pregnancy—and for no rational reason, I predicted that while my first pregnancy might end early, my second would result in a healthy child. But as I gazed out the airplane window, I was struck by a frightening possibility: What if I ended my first pregnancy, then faced the same circumstance on the second? What if I kept conceiving boys with HED? I knew I had a 25 percent chance of conceiving an affected baby with any given pregnancy. But what about conceiving several such sons in a row? Was there a different probability of that happening?

I turned to my math-major husband. "Dan? What are our chances of conceiving a boy with HED twice in a row? Or three times in a row? Is it always 25 percent?"

"No, no," he said, seeing my sudden worry and laying his magazine on the tray table. "It's a simple probability problem. You just multiply."

I looked at him blankly.

"It's like pulling red and blue chips out of a hat, when three quarters of the chips are blue and one quarter are red," he explained. "The first time, you have a 25 percent chance of getting a red. Starting over, you have a 25 percent chance the second time, too. But you only have about a 6 percent chance of pulling reds on both of your first two tries."

It shouldn't have made me feel better, but it did. It was just math—in this case, an attempt to make expectations out of randomness. *Six percent.* I took a false sense of security from that number, letting myself count upon something that could not be counted upon. This was the faith I needed.

Although Dan and I still hadn't written down a plan, we felt more and more like we had made our choice. Test-driving it a little here and there, I took opportunities to talk about it, carefully. As soon as we got to the beach, I began reintroducing myself to Dan's second cousins, whom I had met only briefly at our wedding. A dark-haired woman hurried up to me.

"I'm Gail," she said. "Kayla's mom." Her blond-haired toddler squatted in the sand, digging with real concentration.

"I read your column in *The New York Times*," she said. "What have you and Dan decided to do?"

I was floored by her question. Not even my mother, my sister, or my closest friends had asked me so bluntly. Answering Gail seemed out of the question. But I had only been at the lake for an hour, and I couldn't see shutting down the lines of communication with Dan's family this early in the game. So I stopped stammering, took a deep breath, and took a risk.

"I think we're going to try our luck," I said, still not wanting to reveal too much. I had no idea where Gail's values rested. I had learned enough to know that when strangers asked about our plans, it wasn't always because they cared how our choice suited us. More often, they asked because they wanted to compare our plans to their own experiences or to the path they might take themselves.

A group of water-skiers let out a whoop as they returned to the dock. It was time to set up for the night's barbecue and bonfire. I swallowed through a dry throat and wandered toward Dan's mom, needing someone familiar.

A little while later, as I doctored my hot dog bun, Gail appeared at my side again.

"I am so sorry for asking you such a personal question," she said. "I've just been through so much myself, with fertility treatments and all that, and I consider this an area where I have lots to share. I get excited. I'd really like to talk to you about all of this."

"That's okay," I smiled, getting a better sense of her orientation. "Maybe we can talk some more tomorrow."

The truth was that I didn't want to talk any more about it. I was in a vulnerable, searching place, and Gail was a strong, experienced woman. At that time, I needed a careful listener, not a big sharer. But the next night, at the birthday party, Gail found me as I stood alone, watching boats on the lake as the sun went down.

"What did you mean you were going to 'try your luck'?" she asked.

I was moved by the spirit of the occasion, so against my better judgment, I elaborated.

"We're thinking, at this point, that we'll try to get pregnant on our own. We'll do CVS at about eleven weeks, in order to find out whether our baby is healthy."

"Then what?" she asked, with growing alarm.

Maybe I had misread her. I expected, because of her own experience, that she would support the gamut of women's reproductive rights.

"Well," I said, "then, we'd hope to have a healthy baby. But there's a 25 percent chance that our baby would have HED." I should have stopped, but I wanted to be brave. "So, in that case, we think we'd probably end the pregnancy."

"No!" Her voice was shrill. "You can't do that!"

I looked around, startled. I thought the whole room had heard her. My face burned.

She tried to soften her voice. "Oh my God," she said, "you just can't. We had a surrogate mother for a pregnancy we were trying, and the baby wasn't healthy, so she had an abortion, and it was just *awful*. It was *so* painful for her. She was just crying out, she couldn't believe how much it hurt. I was there. I saw it. You can't do that to yourself. Not physically, and not emotionally."

I stopped hearing her words as she went on. She was antiabortion for *my* sake? I had to admit it was the first time I had heard the perspective that women shouldn't have abortions because it's bad for them.

Gail had been through as many cycles of fertility treatments as anyone I knew, but nothing had worked. Did she still think that was the best option? She seemed to read my question. "You're young and healthy," she said. "The IVF would definitely take."

I wanted to remind Gail that all the drugs and prodding of fertility treatments couldn't have been much better, from a physical perspective, than her surrogate's experience of abortion. I wanted to say that I found it hard to believe that every abortion caused physical agony. It would vary from woman to woman, from provider to provider, and with length of gestation and type of procedure. Anyway, I wanted to tell Gail, physical pain was not my concern; emotional pain mattered more to me. I was trying to have a baby, after all, and childbirth wouldn't exactly be a day at the spa.

But I said nothing.

Dan found me a few minutes later, slouched over a cup of coffee at an empty banquet table.

"Are you crying?" he asked, dropping into the seat next to me. "What happened?"

"I just had a hard conversation," I said, blurting the whole story.

Dan listened with a sympathetic wrinkle in his brow. But his reaction was calm, showing me that he didn't see such tremendous offense.

"It's too bad that happened," he said.

"I'm just seeing that going through all this, trying to get this pregnancy," I said, "it's not going to be easy."

"I know," he said. "Not easy."

He walked me to the car, holding my hand.

Later, I lay in bed too agitated to sleep. My mind seemed to vibrate. The party had overwhelmed me. A dozen cousins had stood and taken turns pouring out appreciation for their great-aunt, for motherhood, for mothers, and mother figures. Blind to the blemishes every family hides, I saw only a big joyful clan, funny little babies, and a great mother figure wizened, forgetful, and revered. Links formed in my mind among family, motherhood, and baby making. As I tried to fall asleep, that trinity made me sad. I knew very well that none of those glowing ideals could create perfect happiness. They were all difficult life journeys, and my own road would be no different.

I replayed my conversation with Gail over and over. Why had I surrendered my integrity, giving her so much influence over my feelings? She was essentially a stranger. I could have dropped her reaction as easily as I dropped my napkin on the table as I left the party. Perhaps in my testing phase, I wanted Gail to play the devil's advocate, to represent one of the many sensibilities my plans could offend. With Gail's help, I was learning what I could handle.

I thought about my resistance to her endorsement of in vitro fertilization. Even removing cost from the equation, something else had me clinging to our new plan. Was I just being selfish, wanting to conceive a baby in the fun way that many of my friends enjoyed? Was I actually willing to sacrifice the nascent life of my own child just to get pregnant as they did in the movies—briefly, easily, privately, and later dancing around the bathroom waving a positive pregnancy test?

Maybe the "normal" way seemed right to me because it offered so much potential for growth, for me personally and for my relationship with Dan. Maybe I wanted to take the opportunity to deepen my character, to see how I would weather something as difficult as a tentative pregnancy. But I checked myself once again. I couldn't get pregnant just to better myself at the possible expense of a fetus. It occurred to me that in order for any option to be painless, I would have to practice detachment from the baby I wanted to grow. But it was too late. I was already attached to the idea of my future baby. I felt I had a particular, biological child waiting to be created and born. And so, every step toward my pregnancy felt intentional and intimate.

In a society where the topic of abortion was typically presented as black and white, I had been marked by the idea that there were only two ways to think about such a choice. We either bestowed on a fetus all the magic of personhood, in which case an abortion would be akin to murder. Or we stripped from the fetus all spirituality and meaning, in which case we would say, "It's just a clump of cells." *But*, I thought as Dan breathed in sleep next to me, *neither of those dogmas seems right.* I tried to articulate a middle place. Even though I didn't believe that pregnancy was miraculous, as people often called it, I did believe it was more special than mere cellular activity. That very cellular activity of pregnancy was remarkable and precious. I realized that until a child became conscious of his own personhood—old enough to recognize and value himself as an individual—other people would bestow his meaning. They would make him special until he could carry himself, and his own sense of worth, into the world.

So, I asked myself, *when shall I decide that my baby is meaningful? Before I conceive? As soon as I know I'm pregnant? After we know he's healthy? Or, as in some cultures, after he is born?* I knew there would be no definitive moment when a zygote, embryo, or fetus inside of me would acquire personhood. My love for the baby would start small and grow along with him. How could I know how tiny or great that love would be by the date of our genetic test—or possible goodbye? It was one of the biggest, scariest unknowns I faced.

Two weeks after our visit to Lake George, I turned twenty-eight. It was the best birthday weekend I could remember. Dan seemed in the mood to celebrate me, so he stretched my birthday into two long, delectable days.

On Saturday, he dropped me off at the bookstore to browse while he drove to the county building to buy a license for our new canoe. Later we visited a rock yard and chose two flat, butterscotch-colored stones. At home, he rolled up his sleeves and did all the grunt work to pound the stones into place: They formed a step between our yard and the neighbor's. Leo and Delia hovered and hopped while we built the step, which provided them a shortcut for their visits. They tested the step every few minutes, and when it was ready—no more wobbles—they ran inside to get their mother.

"I didn't believe it," she said when she came out. "But they were telling the truth. It's wonderful!"

It was an improvement I had envisioned for months, and I couldn't wipe the smile off my face. The more Leo and Delia visited, helping me to fix dinner or brush the cat or plant impatiens, the more our house felt like home. As much as hanging out with kids was a reality check—did I really want to do this all day, every day?—their cheerful voices kept me yearning.

Despite his tired back, Dan was full of energy for an afternoon excursion. We gathered snacks and water, sunscreen and hats, then propped the canoe onto its little two-wheeled trailer. Together we walked down to the lake, finding a shady stretch of flat shoreline from which to launch. We paddled all afternoon, exploring five linked lakes, meandering through canals and neighborhoods. We stopped for tacos at the edge of Lake Calhoun and plowed homeward through a windy chop as the sun dropped. Once we reached Lake Harriet again, we stopped to listen to the last songs of the nightly concert in the band shell. We shared a huge ice-cream cone. Finally, we climbed back into the boat and paddled almost soundlessly home. The sun had set. The water had become smooth and shiny, like melted chocolate. Each droplet from my paddle tip made a perfect doughnut as it pierced the surface. After a full day of work and exercise, I felt calmed by the falling veil of periwinkle twilight. At home with my husband, who had teased and loved me all day as we tracked through the water, I welcomed a long, window-breeze sleep.

The next morning, Dan treated me to a Cuban breakfast in a tiny restaurant cheerfully graffitied down to the last inch. Even though we had stuffed ourselves, he knew well enough to swing by my favorite bakery for éclairs and café au lait. We laughed as we tried to eat the pastries, finding no room in our bellies. We finally decided to pack up our spoils and head to the garden shop. Humoring me, Dan helped me choose tiny mosses and ornamental flowers for the rock garden I wanted to plant in the crevices of the step he had built. At home, as I tucked tiny shoots around the stone steps, I thought about my few years as a gardener. I had proven decent at plotting and sowing, weeding and reaping. I had learned to interpret seed packet instructions for depth, spacing, shade, water. But I knew I was still an amateur, because whenever it came time for thinning—pulling the two smallest of the three sprouts from every hole—I balked. I cringed. I cowered. I stayed inside and washed dishes. I let the summers unwind and allowed my sprouts to grow unchecked. Over and over, I had failed to thin. It always felt too painful and counterintuitive to rip out tiny plants that seemed so viable, so vulnerable. It seemed too great a responsibility to determine, based on appearance alone, which little sprout had the best shot at flowering.

By the time I finished planting, it was only lunchtime. I set to work packing a picnic.

"Kiddo," Dan called from the back porch. "Have you seen this?"

I stepped outside with a block of cheese in one hand and summer sausage in the other. He gently tipped the hanging geranium so I could peer inside. We had seen our pretty red-headed house finches building a nest in the geranium stalks, but this was the first time I had seen their eggs. Sky-blue with rainbow speckles, they looked like Easter-basket candies.

We pedaled to the park and spread our blanket next to Minnehaha Creek to start a long, slow afternoon feast. We took turns slicing cheese and sausage for the bread and eventually tipped onto our backs, spitting cherry seeds into the grass and watching the flight paths overhead.

"DC-9," I said.

A golden retriever walked over our legs.

"Seven-five-seven two hundred," Dan said.

Kids waded ankle-deep in the water.

"A-319 or 20, hard to tell," I said.

It was the same class of aircraft I would take the next morning as I left for Nebraska. I planned to spend most of July there, doing more research and visiting my relatives, including Earl's grave. It had been two years since my last visit.

Dan rested his bare feet on my thighs. "What am I supposed to do around here without you, Kiddo?"

"I hate leaving," I said.

Even though I didn't want to part with Dan, the cat, my blooming gardens, or the tiny blue bird eggs, I felt an urgency about returning to the questions still lingering in my family's past. I wanted to clear my slate of projects; a new one waited on the horizon.

That night, as I fell into bed after packing my bags, I couldn't stop thinking about my age. "I'm twenty-eight," I kept telling myself with the tenor of significance most people reserve for "I'm pregnant." As arbitrary as my plans were, I felt a critical time had come.

The next day, as soon as I was settled into my temporary apartment in Nebraska City, I stepped outside and dialed Aunt Sadie, asking if I could come stay with her for a few days.

"I promise not to ask you a million hard questions this time," I said.

"Well," she responded without finishing. Maybe she did want to share. But I knew her better now, and I felt a soft, protective fondness for her. It felt more important to offer her strength than to squeeze her for stories.

The next morning, I rented a car and began a seven-hour drive to the west. I thought of Dan as I drove, remembering our trip. I recognized the sights; even some bends in the freeway still felt familiar. I felt like Dan was with me, but I also felt alone and inspired. I wasn't certain what I'd find this time, but I knew it would be different.

After a long day's drive, I pulled into Kimball. My first stop was the Co-op Food Store, the same place I'd bought chrysanthemums for Earl's grave on my first visit. After hours in the air-conditioned car, I was startled by the one-hundred-degree heat smothering the parking lot. But I wanted to feel it. Instead of walking directly into the store, I stopped at the little garden center inside a white tent next to the building. There, it was even hotter. The sweet alyssum was overgrown and root-bound. Petunias and geraniums looked vanquished—they wouldn't survive another day of heat like this. I stood still, breathing shallowly. I wanted to soak it up, to feel the heat so deeply that it might help me remember a life that wasn't my own. The far end of the tent offered a small square window of vinyl. The view, framed in searing white, looked like a strange little painting: wavering yellow earth, low and simmering, with train tracks stitching down the horizon. Above, a whistling blue. I wanted to wait there for a train to pass through the painting, but I'd had enough. It was easily 115 degrees in there. Anyway, I had visits to make. Inside the store, I picked up a tiny ivy plant and a bouquet for Sadie.

Just half a mile into town stood the old courthouse. I parked in the shade and walked inside with the little pot of ivy, remembering the feel of the cool, worn steps beneath my sandals. I stepped into the clerk's office, where three ladies—two young, one old—glanced up at me.

"I'm looking for Anita Larson," I said, smiling right at her. "I'm Bonnie. Earl Hickman's granddaughter."

She had already leapt up, with a smile crinkling her face. Reaching over the counter, she pulled me into a hug. She kissed my cheek and looked at me. I pushed the ivy across the counter. Anita looked older than I remembered. But maybe she was only tired. She told me that her husband had been having trouble keeping up with things around the farm, so she was doing all the mowing and hauling and odd jobs herself. And of course, she continued to work at the courthouse, all as she neared her eightieth birthday.

More than anything, Anita was eager for me to hurry along and see Sadie. My great-aunt had turned eighty herself since I had last seen her, and she had recently struggled through a long hospital stay.

"You go see her right now," Anita said, stretching over the counter to hug and kiss me again. "Oh, she'll be so happy to have a visit."

Although the sun had fallen low by the time I arrived at Sadie's doorstep, the air remained a windless one hundred degrees. My great-aunt had been waiting soundlessly, an apparition just behind her screen door. As we hugged, I felt a different energy from her. She seemed happy to see me—giddy, almost, as if her girlfriend had arrived. She sat me on the sofa.

"So," she said. "Your cousins are so excited to see you. We're going out to dinner, then they're going to pick you up. Ryan's softball team needs girls tonight. And later, I have some things to show you. I found a letter that your great-grandmother Josephine wrote to her sister in Washington State, when they were in their early twenties. Before I was born, and before your grandfather. And I've been collecting some things that I think you might like to have. Your grandfather's obituary and a little book of cards people sent when he died. Tomorrow we'll drive out to the farm. I'm guessing you'll want to go out there." She made a soft, strong chuckle. "Am I right?"

All this, and I hadn't asked a single question.

That night under a purple sky, I had three line drive base hits and a handful of RBIs. I had always loved batting, and as a girl, I had loved rough-and-tumble fielding—shortstop especially. But as I got older and taller, I lost my certainty with a glove. Now, I always asked to play right field. My cousin Ryan, a few years younger than I, worked long hours, traded childcare shifts with his ex, and handled his three children kindly and with confidence. The dugout was full of kids—his own, his friends'. I was the oldest woman on the team that night, and the only childless one. I was a strange curiosity to some of the other girls. They offered me beers, laughed with Ryan and their husbands, and tried to figure out what this brainy girl cousin was doing under their ballpark lights.

Ryan's mom, Sarah—Sadie's daughter, a close-in-age cousin to my mother—sat on the wooden bleachers, alternately collecting and releasing her grandkids. I could tell she was watching me, too, pleased to see me taking part instead of simply observing. My camera, which had been affixed to my wrist throughout my previous visit, was now absent. My notepad rested on the nightstand back in the guest room at Sadie's house. Under all those eyes at the softball field, I felt honest and accepted.

Beers cracked for my strong batting, but when I stood in right field, my lack of confidence was obvious. The guys edged closer to me whenever a left-handed batter approached the plate. The game was nearing an end, and we knew we were going to win, when a high fly ball exploded from the bat and careened in my direction. It was dark by then, and the park lights blazed in my peripheral vision. I tried to square up to the ball. Instead of using my instincts to feel my way to a catch as I had done as a girl, I tried to think my way through the motions. *One step back for perspective, just like Dad said. Then go toward the ball. Get underneath it somehow. Get the glove under it—*

There was a resonant thump as the ball cracked into my sternum and plopped to the ground. I didn't fall, but my air was gone. The part I dreaded came next: people running toward me, fit young farmhands, asking urgently if I was okay. I felt a perfectly round bruise spreading between my breasts. It felt as if bits of my windpipe had been smacked loose and splattered high up my throat, blocking my voice. Nothing seemed broken, but for the rest of the evening I could hardly speak.

After the game, as we piled into Sarah's truck with Ryan and his three sleepy children, all I could think about was missing the fly. Why hadn't I caught it? I stood in the perfect position, but I couldn't remember if my glove had even touched the ball. I remembered feeling certain that I would miss. I knew I was capable of catching a fly ball. But I believed I would fail, and so I had.

As my chest ached, I suddenly felt a raw sadness about my

writing, my explorations, my life. What was I doing on a softball diamond in the middle of the wheat fields, a thousand miles from my husband and home? *Should I even be here? What should I be doing?* I wondered as we drove, racing the trains along the highway back to Pine Bluffs.

Driving across the prairie toward Kimball earlier that day, I had spent a good hour talking with my friend Jen, a psychologist, about the dilemma of my genes. I had become obsessed with how other people—even strangers—would judge my choices. I told Jen about my encounter with Gail at Lake George. I shared the experience of an old, close friend almost choking when I told her I might consider abortion. I described my beautiful birthday weekend and my longing to be home with my man-and-cat family. "My mind is eating itself alive," I said. "I'm constantly asking myself what I should do."

"There's your problem," she said. "I try to remind my clients not to ask themselves what they *should* do. Instead, ask yourself what you *want* to do—and then ask yourself how you'll feel if you do it. Your answers are inside of you. Not in someone else's expectations."

A tiny wind, the slightest bit cool, brushed my T-shirt when I climbed out of Sarah's truck. A huge moon had risen over the parched landscape. Inside, I found Sadie wrestling the windows in the guest room, trying to create a cross breeze for me.

As I crawled into bed, I tried Jen's advice.

What do I want? I want to be with Dan. How will I feel if I am with Dan? Loved by my best friend in the world, comfortable, taken care of. Not as independent as I tell myself I want to be. Happy.

Even though it was late in Minneapolis, I called him. "Will you come down here next weekend?" I asked. "I have two weeks left, and I want to spend some time with you in between. Knowing you're coming will help me work harder. And I won't feel so awful about abandoning you in the best part of summer."

"I'll check at work to see if there's room on a flight," he said. I was surprised by how pleased he sounded, how eager to come. I had expected him to tell me that I needed to be working, not playing; his work ethic always outclassed my own. But he said nothing of the sort, and as I hung up the phone, I felt a new lightness: no more guilt and a fresh dose of dizzy love for my husband.

A few parched crickets sang. Tractor trailers whined up the highway, the moon blazed orange, and a handful of fresh molecules swept through the screen and found my skin. Late, I drifted off.

I slept in much too long. The sun was high by the time I came outside to find Sadie watering the flower beds bordering her backyard. We were headed for another bake. It was easily ninety degrees already. Sadie's movements were perfectly even. Each slow sweep of the hose was congruent to the last. She wore long white pants and a blouse. After a lifetime in this climate, she knew how to work without breaking a sweat. I squinted and blinked in the white light. She laughed. "Did you sleep all right?"

I walked with her as she watered and told me the story of each perennial. The garden was simple but flourishing. Some of the plants were huge and old, greening the fence corners and blooming as fully as they could in the wild heat.

"Are you gonna get the car?" she asked. "We should get out to the farm before we all burn up."

I ran the engine until the air conditioner expressed a few cool wisps, then pulled up to the front walk. The hot air made it hard for me to breathe—how could it be safe for the old woman coming down the walkway? I felt as if I were sneaking her out. As we pulled out of town, she wore a little smirk that told me she felt the same way.

To my eye, the Hickman farm had changed little since our last visit. But Sadie seemed pleased with the new tenant. He kept horses on the property, and all four of them stood at the gate when we pulled up to the driveway. I got out and slapped at the animals to get them to stand back. I could hear Sadie laughing in the car. I tried to act tough, to show Sadie the farm stock in me. But I was really a suburban girl, still in love with horses the way a princess-costumed schoolchild would be. I alternated my slaps with long, adoring strokes. How beautiful they were, and how easily I found sentience in their big clear eyes.

Sadie and I retraced our steps around the farmyard. This time, with my combat-reporter guise long gone, she opened up. "You wouldn't have believed the way my mother sang," she told me again, with her hands cupped against the front window of the house. No one was home. "And did you know my dad grew a patch of popping corn for us every year? It was delicious. With real butter."

"I love popcorn," I said. "It's almost a problem. There's no food more comforting to me. Same with my mom."

"Well, now you know where you get it," she said.

Her mind was sharp, perhaps relieved of some of the grief of losing her husband she had been feeling during my first visit. She glanced around the farm, still vexed by its untidiness, but clearly pleased to be back. Her eyes shimmered with memory.

I felt like I was going to faint. How could she stand there like that, in slacks? I wanted to stay longer, but we had to evacuate.

"We should go," I said. She didn't argue.

Back in her kitchen, Sadie pulled open the refrigerator. "We'll have a light lunch," she said. "Since it's so hot, we'll want to save room for supper. Let's make roll-ups." She demonstrated by wrapping a slice of bologna around a stick of string cheese. "And chips and salsa. And I made this Jell-O salad for dinner, but we can taste a little bit now."

I made a mental note about the roll-ups, something to giggle about with Dan later. But eating one wiped the chuckle right off my face. It tasted perfect.

Sadie watched me work my way around my plate. Roll-ups, Jell-O, chips with salsa, then another helping of Jell-O.

"You eat just like my father did," she said. "One thing at a time."

I loved hearing this. Even though I knew Earl had described his father as stern, I couldn't help but appreciate every mossy strand dangling down our family tree.

"I also made us an apple cake," Sadie said, popping up to cut some. "We'll have a little with CoolWhip, and that'll make us look forward to having it again after dinner."

I had to smile. The old gal ate well. She may have been slight, and a little fragile, but she was vigorous.

I had yet to ask Sadie any questions, but I had mentioned the genetic decisions that Dan and I faced—and the fact that we might try for a baby before too many more months went by.

As she finished her cake, she said, "Did I tell you about everything that happened when Jeremy was born?"

I went quiet. Jeremy had been her first child, the one born with HED.

"He came out so dry. So dry I can't describe it. I knew right away that he had it—the condition. It was a hard birth. He was full of fluid because he'd been breech. My parents came to the hospital to help—just in time to see the doctors take him and put him in a hot sunny window to help the fluids go down and keep him warm. Right away I told the doctors, 'No, no, you have to keep him cool.' My parents said the same thing. But they wouldn't listen. I watched my baby there in the window and I knew he needed me. He was too hot. But they wouldn't let me go to him.

"My sister Joan was a nurse, you know. As soon as she saw that boy, she told me to get him down to the children's hospital in Denver. We drove him down, and pretty soon the little guy had IVs and drains all over his poor body, even in his head. It was too much for me. I broke down. I was admitted to the hospital myself. My parents stayed close to the little baby, and he slowly got better. But my parents had seen so much suffering already, watching my brother Earl and my sister Betty struggling with the disorder."

In a stroke of particularly bad genetic luck, Josephine had borne a daughter who was not just a carrier of HED but also suffered from most of the disorder's symptoms—an especially rare circumstance in which the body forms tissues based on the mutated X chromosome instead of the other, presumably healthier, X.

"It bothered my dad in such a deep-down way," Sadie continued. "I think it broke his heart every day to watch those poor kids struggle—his two, and then mine. Little Jeremy would go on to have so many bouts of pneumonia and other things. It was so hard for my dad to see it carry forward into his grandchildren. I remember once when Jeremy was older and I was pregnant again, my father asked me: 'How do you have the courage to have more children?'

"I told him I just never thought about it. I had my next baby, Nathan, and he was healthy. Then I had my two daughters. And I was pregnant again when my dad was getting old and sick."

Sadie stopped and laughed at how quickly I had gobbled my cake. "Do you need some more?"

"No, no," I said, afraid she'd drop the story.

"I'll never forget it," she went on. "My dad was sick. It was February, and I went to the hospital to have my last baby, little Rob. As soon as he heard, my dad came to the hospital to see the baby. I remember the way he looked, coming down the long, long hallway toward me."

Sadie's eyes seemed to be watching her father again: a tired, big-shouldered, bent-backed man shuffling down the corridor.

"He looked so worried," she said. "He came into the room and barely looked at me. He just looked right down into Rob's face, and he breathed the biggest sigh. 'That baby's fine,' he said to me."

Sadie felt that my great-grandfather had held on just to see if the disorder would appear again. Seeing the healthy baby comforted him, and he died three weeks later.

Pausing, Sadie seemed to be somewhere distant for a few moments. Then she said, "It's time for us to take a nap, don't you think?"

This was my kind of woman.

"When we wake up, it'll be time for dinner, and you'll grill the burgers. You can do that, can't you?"

"I think so."

My great-aunt settled upright in her armchair for a snooze, and in the bedroom I fell into my own sticky slumber.

That evening, we chattered like old girlfriends. A breeze picked up. A few clouds formed strips on the horizon—a promise of cool to come. I undercooked the burgers, but Sadie ate hers anyway, not exactly insisting that it was delicious. All I could do was laugh; guilt, apology, or a second try would be too much effort on an evening so stifling hot. As the sun dropped low and lit the arriving clouds pink, Sadie finished a second round of apple cake and CoolWhip. Then she said, "Let's go for a ride."

She drove me up the bluff, showing me the farm where she and Uncle Stanley had lived as newlyweds. Riding along, I could see the rocky outcrops where my mother must have explored the bluff as a girl. Being in Sadie's air-conditioned car was respite enough, but there was something especially soothing about swooping downhill as we turned back toward Pine Bluffs.

Just as we reached the edge of town—a barely perceptible transition from farm country to gridded streets—Sadie slowed the car. "I thought I'd show you where they're going to plant me," she said, glancing over. "If you want to see."

"I'd like to."

She turned in to the small cemetery where her husband and two sons lay buried. Her husband, Stan, had been there for just over two years. Jeremy, the eldest, rested next to his brother. Both of them had been gone for decades, having died in their early twenties.

"They were best friends," Sadie said of her first two children. "I think about them every day." She looked at me, as if to make sure I understood: *every day*.

Nathan, her second son, had seen a breakdown on the side of the highway one snowy night. He pulled over to help. When he stepped out of the car, a truck hit him.

A few years before that, Jeremy, her boy with HED, had returned home from college for the summer. On a hot day, a local farmer hired him and another young man from Kimball to help build a new silo. With a wet T-shirt under his leather jacket, Jeremy rode his motorcycle to work. First, the farmer needed help moving huge sheets of metal across the farmyard to the site of the new outbuilding. With one of the panels propped on his tractor, the farmer drove slowly. The two young men walked along each side, holding the giant sail steady. But no one thought to look up; the farmer drove the metal sheet into a power line. The whole thing electrified, snapping Jeremy to death right away and burning the other worker gruesomely.

"I always wondered," Sadie told me, "if that wet T-shirt made the difference."

The news came in a phone call taken by little Sarah. She told her mother Jeremy had been in an accident, but couldn't say more. Sadie piled the kids into the car with no idea where to drive. She cried and panicked, careening through the country-side, looking for signs of her firstborn son in field after field. When she finally found him, Stanley was already at his side. The priest had administered last rites. The farmer stood, hat in hand. No one had moved Jeremy's body from the place it fell. They all felt his mother should touch him first.

"Here," Sadie said, gesturing from the car window. "I'll be next to Stan. With the boys right at our side."

* * *

The next morning, driving east again and soon to see Dan, I stopped again at the Co-op Food Store to pick up one more bunch of fresh flowers. Then I drove to the Kimball Cemetery.

I found my grandfather's grave quickly this time. The scene was so familiar that I could have sworn I'd gone back in time. Sprinklers chucked, barely doing the job as the sun quickly dried every drop from every blade of grass. The same dawn-colored mourning doves walked near the spray, jockeying for a drink. Flags whipped above me, a rooster crowed from the yard of a nearby house, and a train rumbled past, dividing earth from sky.

Standing alone with my grandfather, I felt reassured. His story was part of my own. I was carrying forward the stories folded into me at birth. I would make of them whatever I could. The decision I was making with Dan was a decision only for us, in our family, in our moment. I knew in many ways it was a fallacy to use my grandfather's life story to influence our choice, but we belonged to the same family, to the same narrative. And those stories would continue to exert forces on our family tree, however each generation might interpret them. Were lives with HED worth living? I couldn't even pretend such a question should exist. In each family, in each branch of lineage, for each individual mother and father, the answer was unique.

I hadn't planned to speak to my grandfather, but as I stood there, words sprang up. "I know more about how you got here." The sound of my voice startled me. It reminded me how alive I was and made me feel solitary. "I know more about what happened. I still have to use my imagination a lot, though," I said, as if to ready him for difficult news.

Sadie had been keeping watch over everyone. Her parents, as well as all of her siblings buried there, had bouquets of silk flowers secured in vases on their headstones. I carried my own fresh bouquet, along with a bottle of water I had intended to pour into Earl's vase. But his silk flowers were lodged so tightly that I wouldn't be able to get them out without tearing them. And what would I do with them if I did get them out? I couldn't very well bring them back to Sadie. So instead, I unwrapped the blooms I'd brought: statice, daisies, cushion mums. One by one, I laid the stalks across the length of my grandfather's grave.

The sun had begun to sear my neck and arms, but I sat down next to him and twined my fingers through the grass, down to the soil. Remembering the magnetism I'd felt on my first visit to him, I was surprised by how thin my grandfather's presence seemed now. He felt less alive, less mysterious, and less needful.

"I turned twenty-eight last week," I told him. "Dan and I want to get pregnant this fall."

I stopped. I had never described our plans, with any certainty, out loud before—even to myself. My voice began to wobble.

"If we find ourselves pregnant with a little boy with HED, we plan to . . . have an abortion."

The sun heated the tears on my face, making them feel like they belonged to someone else. "It's not because we wouldn't love and adore him and cherish his presence in our lives." I stopped, feeling stuck. I wanted to explain our choice in terms of the reasons we *had* used, not the reasons we hadn't. I sat for a long time, searching. And finally my head came up.

"You don't need me to explain," I said. "You understand better than anyone."

I stood up and uncapped the water I had brought for the flowers. It glugged softly as I poured it over him, from his head to his toes, cold and wet and plentiful.

Back in the car, I pawed through my bags until I found paper and a pen. Scribbling as quickly as I could, I recorded everything. I couldn't wait to see Dan. I needed to tell him that our decision was safe. I had finally written it down.

paula

After my dad came home from Mount Airy, there was no money. He scared us. He was afraid someone would kidnap us. I remember walking home from school through the park after he warned us not to talk to strangers. I made up a fake language and kept jabbering it as loud as I could and swinging my arms all over the place. I made myself look like a lunatic. None of my friends would even walk with me anymore. But I figured kidnappers wouldn't want a crazy person.

At school, we lined up to visit the fourth-grade classrooms and get a preview of the coming year. The staff had a long list they read out loud, telling us which teacher we would have. Everybody wanted Mrs. Duncan. She had big soft wrinkles in her face and pretty brown eyes, and she loved to sing and do melted-crayon art and she would put her hand so softly on our heads when we went by. I never won anything, so when they read the list, I was so surprised: "Paula Hickman, Mrs. Duncan." I ran home fast that day—straight and sane but faster than kidnappers—to tell my mom I would have Mrs. Duncan for fourth grade in the fall. "Oh, Paula," she said, and she just hugged me. She seemed sad, like there was something she couldn't say. By the last day of school, I was putting the pieces together. My aunt Sadie had been on the phone with my dad a lot. I heard him telling my mom, "It's a nice house straight across the street from her and Stan and the kids in Pine Bluffs."

"What are you going to do?" my mom asked him.

"I'll be close to the pharmacies in Casper and Kimball and not too far from Cheyenne either, and I'm looking into opening a pharmacy in Pine Bluffs, too. Lots of opportunities."

"Can we afford the house?"

"It's a rental," he told her.

Her face fell, and he said, "There is no shame in that."

That time, I was actually on my dad's side. I liked it when he tried to keep my mom down to earth. But now I think she must have just realized that everything they'd put into the house in Greeley was gone.

They would tell us things about how much we were going to love it in Wyoming. "It's going to be so nice in Pine Bluffs," my mom would say. "You can play with your cousins every day, and there's a huge rock cliff you can climb all over—that's the bluff. But you have to watch out for rattlesnakes, you know. If you be careful, it'll be fun like cowboys."

We were all in the car with everything we could take with us, and it was a hot summer day, and as my dad backed down the driveway we were all staring straight ahead at our empty house. I had a bad feeling. Greg was quiet and Curt was talking baby talk. The bad feeling told me that it wasn't going to be better in Pine Bluffs. It was going to be worse. My mom and dad weren't talking to each other in the front seat. The lake was going by, and I started crying, and I just blurted out, "But I have to have Mrs. Duncan next year!"

My mom just kept her face forward and said, "Listen, Paula, you might as well stop crying. We can't stay here."

* * *

In Pine Bluffs our neighbor let me ride her horse, Blaze, up the bluff. Once I was climbing around on the rocks way above her yard, and I heard a rattlesnake. I screamed down to her, "Snake! Snake!" She was in her garden, and she picked up a rock and said, "When it hits, you run down!" She threw the rock and it clattered against the cliff and distracted the snake. I ran all the way down, getting gravel in my shoes. It was one of the first times when I was scared but also felt brave and tough. Soon I learned how to shoot a rifle and a bow and arrow.

My dad didn't have a job. He said he was looking for one. So right when we got there, that summer, he spent some extra time with us. Our new house had a wagon-wheel fence, and I think that gave him the idea for how to decorate our bikes for the summer parade. He called it "Pine Bluffs Past, Pine Bluffs Present." We took the cardboard boxes from moving and cut them up, and my dad bent them into a huge pointed rocket and made it shoot up from my handlebars. Then we had red streamers for the blastoff hanging down over my wheels. I wore Greg's astronaut helmet, and I was The Present. For Greg's bike, we used our hula hoops and draped a sheet over them to make a covered wagon and even painted a little brown buffalo onto the side. I had no idea my dad could make such a real-looking buffalo. Greg wore a cowboy hat and his boots, and he was The Past. At the end of the parade, the lady said Greg and I won first and second place to share.

It was one of the coolest things our dad ever did with us. I think that's why I always made such a big deal of you kids decorating your bikes for Derby Days in Redmond. Remember when you pulled your sister in the wagon behind your trike, and you were the tortoise and the hare? And the time we made your bike into a hot-air balloon? When my dad decorated the bikes with us, it was one of the last times I really knew he loved us. I think he felt that, too. He was so proud of himself. He kept talking to my mom about everything he'd done and how much we loved it.

She didn't build him up. He was jobless, and more and more he just slept on the couch. Every few days he'd have a new idea or project or some old thing he wanted to start working on again, but she had learned not to get her hopes up. Instead she was looking around, trying to figure out what she could do for work, if my dad could just stay home with Curt while Greg and I were at school. But she was a nurse and there was no hospital in Pine Bluffs. There wasn't even a doctor's office. My dad said he was going to start a pharmacy so people who had to go all the way to Kimball to see the doctor could still get their prescriptions refilled in their own hometown. Sometimes he made lists of the drugs he wanted to stock—he said he wanted "classy drugs for classy people." They were probably just all his favorite ones.

One day we were across the street at Aunt Sadie's, and I was supposed to be playing with my cousins, but I heard my mom and aunt in the kitchen. Nobody ever argued with Aunt Sadie, so I went down the hall to see what was going on. I heard my mom saying, "Well, if only your mother hadn't coddled him so much!" and that made Sadie so angry.

I don't know where he went during the daytimes, but when I think back on the days when he wasn't just sleeping on the couch, he did leave the house. At night when he came home, he still came to my bedside and would say, "I love you, my little Baby Doll," like he always had. He would kiss my cheek and put his hand on my head. I had gotten good at keeping still and pretending to be asleep. But it got even harder not to open my eyes in those days, because I could tell he was crying.

I asked Greg if he ever said "I love you" to Dad. He said he didn't, and I said, "Me neither." I was getting afraid to.

"Let's practice," I said to Greg. "You pretend I'm Dad, and you say it first."

"I love you."

"Not so fast."

"I love you."

"No, say it slow, like you mean it. I. Love. *You*. Like that."

We took turns trying it, and we kept practicing together all the time.

I really felt sorry for my dad. It seemed like my mom was wearing him down. I asked her, "Mom, why are you making Dad sad? How come you keep making him cry?"

I thought all they needed was to be more lovey with each other, like they had been in Broomfield. Now, when they fought, they went right up toe-to-toe. She would scream at him, "How can you say it like that to me, Earl? To my face? The loan hasn't come through *yet*. Right to my face like that! You lie too easily, much too easily!"

It was normal for Mom to raise her voice—she was always shaping us up that way. But my dad was always so sleepy and hoarse and tired that I hardly ever heard him yell. Even when he did, his voice was so much quieter than hers. But it scared me more. I yelled, too: "No, Mom! No, Dad! Stop it! No fighting! Hug! Hug each other!" But I don't think they could even feel me down there, trying to push their bodies together.

When my mom yelled in whispers, then I knew it was especially bad. Dad was sleeping on the couch every time the owners came to collect the rent. "How am I to tell your sister that you haven't paid their friends a penny?" my mom would say after she closed the door. "I am so ashamed."

My dad was impossible to wake up. In Greeley, if we jumped on the bed long enough, he'd wake up. But in Pine Bluffs, Greg and I were bigger, and there wasn't room to jump on the couch. Still, we tried sometimes. "Dad! Daaad!" We would bounce around like crazy, but it was like he could sleep through a storm and sink in a ship and never even know what happened.

He wouldn't wake up to go to church with us on Sundays. I

sat there in church looking around. Dads with brown hair. Dads with black hair. Dads like mine with only a little hair. Dads with gray hair. Dads with curly hair. Dads in red shirts, dads in blue shirts, dads in white shirts, and lots of skinny, long ties. Dads in suits. Dads carrying babies. Dads holding hands. Holding hands with moms. Holding hands with their kids. Shaking hands with the priest and the altar boys and all the other dads.

At our new school, my teacher put on a movie. She said we were to watch it and learn the risks we ran. She said, "Sometimes people take drugs, and then they can't stop. So you must make good choices." It didn't mean anything to me at first, but then the movie started—it was called "Dick Smith: Drug Addict"—and everything hit me. The guy was using heroin, and he tried to stop when he was in jail, but he still couldn't. He couldn't stop because it hurt him too much, and he kept banging his head on the cell wall. Then he was dead and looking back and telling how his life fell apart, how he once had a family and a job and everything was good, but then the drugs made him go crazy and sleep all the time and make no sense. He crashed into things at night and slept on the couch in the daytime—or just wherever he fell down—and he couldn't work and he couldn't play with his kids. At the part where he just wouldn't get up, not for his kids or anything, my face got boiling hot. I just put my head down on my desk and wrapped my arms around my ears. Blood was pounding in my head, and I just kept thinking, *Now everyone knows.*

We hadn't been in Pine Bluffs for a year before my mom had to go to work, so we moved to Cheyenne where there was a hospital. The house had cardboard walls and bats in the basement. My mom always made me be the one to go down to the basement to get the ice cream from the freezer. She said she was too tall and her hair would tangle with the bats. I didn't even like ice cream. I hated going down there, and then I'd have to run back up the stairs so scared I couldn't breathe while they flapped around me.

My dad thought we were far enough from Greeley that his creditors wouldn't find him. Whoever they were. But one night my dad jumped up and said, "Lock the doors, Esta. Quick!"

"Go to your rooms!" my mom yelled. Curt was already in his bed, but Greg ran to his room and I ran to mine, where I could look out the window to the driveway.

"Don't look outside," my dad said to my mom in the living room. "I mean it! Don't watch!" But from my room, I watched. I could see everything. It was dark out there, but I could see the car my dad was afraid of. It was a dark car, black. They turned their lights off when they pulled into the driveway. They hardly said anything. My dad pulled off his sweater and there was all this scraping and shuffling from their feet in the gravel. I heard my dad go *uh, whff.* I don't know why I didn't scream. I just couldn't. I saw my dad sitting down on the ground, on his knees. The men walked away, back to the car, and backed up until they were under the streetlights and drove away. I watched my dad crawl around in the gravel. He found his glasses and blew on them. Then he found his teeth and brushed them on his pants and put them back in his mouth.

In the living room my mom screamed at him and cried with this terrified kind of fury. He kept saying, "I'm sorry about that, Esta. I'm so, so sorry they came to our house. But I promise they won't be back. I broke at least one nose out there. They won't be bothering us anymore. Come here. Shh. Sh."

In the daytime, my mom worked and my dad slept. When it was late in the fall and too cold to play outside after school, I just stared out my dirty bedroom window at the gray old weeds blowing around outside. I tried praying. *Please God, please God. Please make it better. Make my dad better and make our parents love us. Make my dad wear his suit and mow the lawn for that sweet smell like he did when we were little. Make all those weeds stop swirling around in the wind. Make it warm and nice out there.*

Next door was Joey, and he was my best friend for a little while. We loved to dance in his living room. It was the most fun I remember from that time, just dancing around his living room with the most serious looks on our faces, concentrating so hard on how it felt to let go.

I got my dad to drive the two of us to the movies. *Goldfinger* was out. We were riding in the backseat and Joey said, "What the heck is your dad doing with that little bottle?"

"What little bottle?"

He pointed up at my dad. All I could see was the back of his head, so I looked around the seat and saw what Joey meant. My dad had a little soft plastic bottle of model airplane glue, and he was holding it right under his nose. He kept squeezing it a little, puffing it up into his nostrils.

I told Joey I didn't know what it was. I said, "Dad, stop doing that, okay?" Then I looked at Joey and said, "Haha."

Later when I was in the car with Dad and Greg, I asked my brother, "What's Dad doing with that bottle?"

Greg looked around the seat just like I had before. He said, "Dad, quit doing that bottle sniffing when you're driving us. Our friends are gonna see you and think you're a druggie. *Dad.*"

But it was like he couldn't even hear us. He had a little soft smile on his face, like he thought we were cute. It seemed like he was just in love with the song on the radio and pleased as punch with us kids in the backseat. He was happy as a clam, a sniff-sniffing clam.

Once, when they delivered the coal, bats flew up out of the basement into the house. I screamed and screamed, and my dad woke up and jumped off the couch and came into the kitchen going "What? What, Paula?" He saw the bats and chased them all out.

Later I did more of that same screaming in my room. I screamed like it was a kind of wild dance music. I wanted to bring him back, to wake him up and keep him awake. But when he came to my room that time, he just looked tired. He didn't even spank me for crying wolf. Mom was the only one who bothered to spank us anymore, and she was always working. I just went outside. I played around for a while in our yard and finally knocked on the door at Joey's house. Nobody answered even though I could hear them in there. It was happening more and more like that.

There was a paved part between the houses. I played jacks there forever, until the sun went down and I had to find something to eat. Other times I would draw huge hopscotch grids for myself and tiny ones for fairies and leprechauns. Our big dog Prince would lay out there with me and walk with me out on the road. I always knew if I fell and broke my leg or got beat up or hit by a car, he would hang me softly in his mouth and carry me home.

The first night it happened, I woke up with my heart beating so fast. There was banging and the walls rumbled. "Mom! What is that? What is that crashing?" I could hear them out in the hall, my mom and my dad, her whispering loudly with him. I could barely hear him at all. Just his little scrapy breaths. In the morning she told me it was my dad who made the noises. He couldn't see too well at night, and his feet pounded too hard when he tried to get down the hall to the bathroom, or some weird excuse like that. He ran into the wall, she said, and it was just an accident. But I had seen the movie at school. I knew why. It was only the first time of many. When he crashed around at night, it shook the whole house. My heart would pound so hard. Out in the hallway when she tried to collect him and bring him back to bed, my mom would say, *Uch, ick!* She hated the matted dirty carpet and thin rattling walls and blamed them.

Almost every weekend, Aunt Sadie came fifty miles from Pine Bluffs to Cheyenne to get us kids. She took us back to Pine Bluffs to play on the rocks and see our cousins and have normal days. Once, when we got into her car, she started the engine and shook her head.

"What?" I asked.

She shook her head again—she didn't like to speak out of turn, my mom always said. But then she did. "I don't know how you can live in that place," she said.

We had one Christmas in that house in Cheyenne. I got pink curlers in my stocking. I couldn't wait to do my hair. I had this long, pretty blond hair. Everybody at school was always saying I had the prettiest hair in fifth grade. Now I could even curl it.

My dad said, "Close your eyes, Esta."

He went over into the kitchen and there was the sound of a cardboard box scraping across the linoleum floor and into sight. It had a huge red bow. He pushed it into the living room next to the tree, right in front of Mom's knees, and he said, "Merry Christmas."

I couldn't believe it. She couldn't believe it either. She opened her eyes and let out her breath—a dishwasher! "Earl, thank you," she said. In the kitchen he showed her how the hose hooked up to the sink and how it wheeled away into the corner when she didn't need it. She said, "Mm-hm," as she listened. Then she bent by his ear and said, "Earl, how much did this cost? You need to tell me exactly so I can balance the checkbook." Then she stood up and pushed her hands down her skirt and said, "Ah, this is the nicest Christmas gift ever. What a happy Christmas, eh kids?"

It was. But then things got weird again. A few days later, my dad talked me into driving back to Pine Bluffs with him so his sister Betty could cut my hair at her beauty shop. My mom kept telling me not to listen to him, not to do it. Now I have to wonder if he wanted to sell my hair or something. Betty always wore a wig because of the disorder—maybe she knew where he could send my hair for cash. Or maybe he just wanted an excuse to see his family and ask to borrow more money. But he somehow convinced me that it was a good idea, so we went, and I ended

up with plain straight hair just past my ears. When I went back
to school, everybody asked, "Oh, Paula, where's all your pretty
hair?" It was so short, I couldn't get a single one of my pink
curlers to stay in.

We lived a long bus ride from school. In the year we lived
in that house, only once did a girl from school come over. I got
really good at jacks, hopscotch, talking to my dog—things I
could do alone.

earl

Esta's paychecks sustained us in Cheyenne. I worked at my desk when I could.

"Everything will resolve," I told her. "My dreams and yours."

"I am sick of the way I believe in you like God," she said.

Debt returned in a night visit. It was a resurgent account, a loan seemingly forgiven but arisen again, monstrous, fat-fisted, coming to my home to harm my children, to scour their little wide eyes.

I thought I would try something new. Mode O'Day stores were growing, and I wanted to open a franchise in Cheyenne. Everything should have worked, but the timing was off. There was no immediate profit to cover the check I wrote for my stock. It was a big check and worthless. They arrested me at my front door, in front of my children. My daughter frozen there with her schoolbag, the last bite of cereal still in her mouth. They took my teeth when they booked me. I only spent three days in jail, but when I returned, by the way Paula sobbed with hatred and relief, I could see she thought she had lost me for the last time.

When Sadie came out from Pine Bluffs to take the children one weekend, she said to me, "Our cousin Ethel found a job for you in Seattle. A respiratory therapist, for West Seattle General Hospital." She made me look into her eyes. "Earl, take your sweet little ones and your precious wife and go. This will be a fresh start. A regular job with regular hours and a regular employer. No more projects. No more enterprises. It's because of your Nebulizer, you know. They agreed to hire you because you know all about respiration and delivering medicines to the lungs. You were made for this. All of your accomplishments led right up to it, and now you have arrived. I am so proud of you. We all are, you know."

"Esta," I said later to my wife, "no one will judge us. No one has to know. It is the last thing we need to do before we can start over. That is the purpose of bankruptcy provisions. You keep saying it yourself: *We need a fresh start.* Well, here it is. No one will bother us anymore. None of this follows us to Seattle."

But she cried and cried and felt so ashamed.

I returned from Nebraska to Minneapolis in the middle of a sickening late July heat wave. With no air conditioning, historic humidity, and blazing temperatures starting each morning in the nineties and climbing from there, I could focus on nothing else. Our hairy cat staggered around, moaning like a drunk. I pined for a window unit, while Dan, always one for a challenge, was oddly spirited. We had been sleeping at night with phonebook-size ice packs inside our pillowcases. Dan kept telling me to try to make it just a few more days, but he knew he'd lost the battle when he found me crying in the basement.

"Get me out of here," I whined.

He smiled at the opportunity for an adventure, then sprang upstairs to pull up a radar map on the computer.

"Okay, Kiddo," he said a few minutes later. "Stay down here where it's cool until you know exactly what you want to run upstairs and pack. I'll have the car running with the A/C on. We're going north. There's a storm cloud over Brainerd."

He sealed our bins of camp gear, dumped a cascade of ice and drinks and snacks into the cooler, and loaded the car. I dragged myself upstairs to stuff a backpack. We put ice in all of the cat's water bowls and asked the neighbors to keep watch in case he passed out.

Half an hour later, in the cool car, Dan was relieved to find me cheerful again. Extreme heat had always made me a monster. I thought of my brother and grandfather, who as far as I knew managed to keep from throwing tantrums on hot days. Perhaps their survival instincts were stronger than mine; they had no energy to waste on grumbling.

We spun north for two hours, and there we found it: a massive bank of storm clouds with a tail so long that it promised to keep us cool all night. When we reached our campground, I timidly rolled down a window and stuck out my arm.

"Roll 'em all down," Dan said. The air temperature had dropped a good thirty degrees, and there was a cool jitter in the atmosphere.

Dan built a fire while I fried sausages and sliced tomatoes for dinner. Refreshed, I chattered about the fertility chart I had begun keeping as I tracked my monthly cycle. Taking my temperature each morning and watching my body's signs, I was beginning to understand my pattern, which would be useful when we decided it was time.

It obsessed me to imagine my ovaries and uterus preparing themselves in the normal way for the possibility of a pregnancy. Assuming my birth control pills had always done the trick, I hadn't ovulated in ten years. I was transfixed by the idea that I would actually release an egg within a day or two.

"I should have fertile fluid either today or tomorrow," I said with a dramatic suggestive tone. "We could try, if you wanted to."

"Getting pregnant is all you can think about," Dan said, coaxing his fire, keeping his gaze away from mine.

His words had an air of challenge. But he was certainly right. So I stuffed the defensive little burn that rose in my throat. "I know," I said, wiping my knife with a paper towel. "I guess I've just spent these last years preparing. Looking toward this fall.

Here it is almost August, which is almost fall, and I'm done preparing. I feel ready."

"We don't *have* to start trying this fall, though," he said. "I mean, just think how much more of this we could do." He gestured toward the river, which we had just finished exploring in an afternoon of muddy bank scrambles and camera flashes and hurled rocks. "And our flight benefits are amazing," he went on. "You still want to go to Africa, don't you? And we haven't been to China or India, and we always thought we'd go to South America before we started a family."

I could barely hear him. Blood pumped in my ears. I had heard myself say, *I'm ready*, and now it was all I could think.

"Can we try this week?" I asked him point-blank, deaf to everything he'd been saying.

"No," he said.

I jumped a little, unaccustomed to power struggles like this. "What do you mean? Then when?"

"It's not fall yet," he said. "I don't even know if this fall is a good idea anymore. We're going into debt; how are we going to afford a baby? You always say you don't want to be working outside the house when we have a baby. I don't see how we're going to do it." He sighed and turned back to the fire. The sky darkened with a welcome stormy promise.

"Don't you see what I'm asking?" he finally asked. "What about *us*?"

I began to cry. My tears alarmed him more than they should have. I had been a waterspout of late. I cried when I read the spines of the books in the pregnancy and parenting section at the bookstore. I cried when I thought about the foods I would eat to nourish a baby during pregnancy. I even cried when I happened to see a random Internet post about the maternal beauty of a woman's postpartum body.

"It's going to be so hard," I croaked as the fire spat into the air. "I just know that once I'm pregnant, I'm going to experience the hardest three months of my life while we wait for those test results. And you know me," I said, looking for his eyes in the firelight. "You know the way I always want to meet a challenge right away, instead of putting it off."

My husband sat quietly, nudging the burning logs with a bone-white stick.

"I don't know, Kiddo," he said. "I still think we have so much youth left. I know I always said I wanted to have a baby by the time I was thirty—"

"And you'll be thirty-one in a month."

"But I feel like we have more time," he said. "There's more to explore."

The day before, we had gone to a mall bookstore for relief from the heat. Right away, I had dragged Dan over to the pregnancy section. "Well," I said, seeing how he squirmed, "if you don't want to look, then can I at least choose a few for you?"

"That's fine," he answered, hurrying off. Half an hour later, I found him crouching between two high shelves, with a globe's worth of travel guides spread around him.

Now, our campfire drew down. "It's almost too much," I said. "The thought of getting pregnant—pulling that off—and then undoing it. I feel brave right now. Just brave enough. I'm afraid I'll lose my courage if we wait too long."

"We don't *have* to stick with our plan for the testing," Dan said. I was surprised.

"Yes, we do," I said, surprising myself. I had been poring over my grandfather's medical records. I had found and interviewed two of his old doctors, and, following their leads, dug even more deeply into the medical literature on HED. So many of Earl's tribulations had passed through my hands in recent months—court orders, restraining orders, divorce papers, bankruptcy proceedings, hospitalizations—blow after blow, all leading up to his death certificate.

"We should stick with it," I said. "But it's going to be hard."

Dan turned to me. "Maybe it won't be as hard as you think," he said. "We can't go through those first three months thinking things will go wrong. That doesn't make any sense. We should be preparing ourselves for a baby, not a tragedy." He watched the embers as he stirred them.

Before we crawled into the tent, we decided to pull off the rain fly so we could watch the clouds alternate with stars as the wind cooled our sticky skin. Our tired eyelids peeled open with the night's biggest lightning flashes. Here and there, we welcomed little rain spatters onto our legs, arms, and faces. After days of no-touch heat, we lay motionless on our backs with our sides pressed together. Nothing made sense, but I felt like I was home.

Into August Dan and I met weekends with new urgency. We combed our city parks, paddled our lake, and tried all of our neighborhood restaurants. We flew to Boise to see friends and to Vermont to explore the late-summer countryside. One night, with just a few days left in August, I skewered pork for Dan to grill. He sat at the table, resting after mowing the lawn and pulling weeds. Leo and Delia squawked in their backyard, brandishing water guns.

"I'm going to be fertile again next week," I said to Dan.

He made a small, anguished sound.

"What?" I asked, indignant.

"It's just the travels," he said. "We haven't even taken our canoe up to the Boundary Waters. I've never really been on a backpacking trip with you in the mountains. I still want to learn to ski. I haven't shown you the Grand Canyon. There's so much we still have to do."

I kept my mouth shut and slowly washed lettuce. There was no reason to think we would stop living once our child was born. And aside from that, I thought, it was crazy to think we would have enough time in our lives to see the whole planet anyway or learn everything it had to offer. When would he feel he had seen and done enough to become a father? His objection could hold forever.

In our silence, he had the same thought. I turned to see him drop his forehead to the table, hiding his face inside his folded arms. "I don't really know what I'm waiting for," he moaned. "How many places would I have to go before I'd feel ready?"

Treading carefully, I said, "Maybe this month, we could just try for a girl. The chances of conceiving are smaller if we do that. If it doesn't work, we'll have more time. It's a win-win."

There were ways, I had learned, to increase our chances of conceiving a girl, in which case our child would either be entirely HED-free or simply a carrier like myself. We knew that sperm determined the sex of a baby. Researchers had figured out that sperm carrying female chromosomes are slower and tougher than sperm carrying male chromosomes. In other words, girls were the tortoises, boys were the hares. So, to conceive a girl, we had to time intercourse for three or four days before my ovary would release an egg—then, no more sex until the fertile period passed. That way, by the time an egg tumbled down, any surviving sperm still waiting around would most likely be female. It would certainly be a bit of a guessing game, since an egg's release could be delayed by any number of factors. Or, I might misread my body's signs and time sex too close to ovulation, in which case we'd be more likely to conceive a son.

Even though the odds were better, conceiving a girl would not be fail-safe in terms of HED. There was the remotest chance that she could be born with the major symptoms of HED, as my grandfather's sister Betty had been.

"There is no data on that," our new genetic counselor said when I called to ask about the chances that our daughter could suffer from fully expressed HED. But she didn't offer to hunt for an answer. I remembered Virginia Sybert, the gentle doctor in Seattle who had known my brother since he was a newborn and who examined me before I knew I was a carrier. I sent her an e-mail and asked her to estimate the chances of conceiving an affected female. She responded the next day, saying that her research led her to guess that for a carrier, the chances of actually exhibiting the disorder might be 5 percent. Even though there was no way to differentiate, with in utero testing, a healthy carrier female from an affected carrier female, Dan and I felt we could accept that risk since the chances were so minimal. Finding out I was pregnant with a girl, whether or not she carried HED, would be good news: We would keep our pregnancy.

Even if she didn't suffer from HED, our daughter would have a 50 percent chance of someday being faced with the dilemma of whether, and how, to avoid passing HED to her own children. I wondered, *Would she think I had been callous about the decisions I faced? Would she find me embarrassingly freethinking? If she found out her mother had undergone an abortion, would she be ashamed? Would she mourn?* Maybe my daughter would not be the type to contemplate any of these things. Maybe she would blissfully become pregnant one day, never for a moment considering the old stories to which her mother clung. I imagined her marking a new beginning in the chain of inheritance I wanted to break. Yet I knew, no matter what I preferred, that these would be her choices.

At the same time, I assumed that two decades into the future, my daughter might have less expensive and less painful options than mine. A test might be able to reveal, after only a few weeks' pregnancy, whether she carried a baby with the disorder. Such an early test would limit the duration of a tentative pregnancy, permitting a seemingly less complicated abortion.

Scientists had recently cured fetal mice of HED by injecting genetic material through the womb, actually correcting the errors in their DNA. Could humans benefit from the same procedure by the time my daughter might decide to become a mother? Perhaps she would be able to become pregnant the natural way and still be guaranteed, with some medical help, a healthy baby. But she might face other challenges, I thought. Would my legal right to an abortion survive into my daughter's era?

A few days later, Dan and I both knew the unspoken: Our window was opening, and I had less than a week until ovulation.

"What do you think about trying?" I asked tentatively one night as we undressed.

"We can try," he said. His tone was even. He folded his clothes into a drawer as I looked for his eyes in the dim light. He glanced over at me and nodded, as if to say he was sure.

We had heard about the Minnesota State Fair, and since we had been in the business of exploring, we knew we needed to check it out. I found cheap tickets for a Tuesday evening and picked Dan up from work. It was warm, with a sky awash in orange. A mass of people shape-shifted over the grounds, thickening between barns, clustering around rides, and clotting at food booths. We marveled at individuals eating entire bucketfuls of warm chocolate-chip cookies, and others who moved through the crowds with Pronto Pups in one hand and deep-fried Twinkies in the other. We did our best to fit in, sharing lamb on a stick, hot dog on a stick, walleye on a stick, even casserole on a stick. "Gotta do it," we said, grinning, every time we added a new delicacy to the bellyaches we were seeding. Dan had to try the Tom Thumb mini donuts, so in solidarity, I dipped into the bag as well. Then we guzzled homemade birch beer and split an order of strawberry shortcake. Stuffed and slow, we wandered through the exhibition halls, checking out carriage-size pumpkins and roomfuls of blazing gladiolus. In the Miracle of Birth barn, we watched a cow licking her newborn calf. We giggled at the newly hatched chicks spinning on a miniature Ferris wheel. On our way out, we passed a ewe huffing through labor, ignoring the gaggle of children clamoring around her.

The sky darkened, and Dan bought us tickets for the Ferris wheel. When we stepped up to the platform, the attendant asked us how we felt about sharing our cart with another couple.

"We'll wait for our own," Dan said.

I was thankful, as we watched the ride spin, that Dan wanted to be alone with me. We hadn't spoken a word about our pregnancy attempt a few nights before, and neither of us had gone out of our way to create a quiet moment to connect. With so much unspoken, I was surprised by how nervous I felt when the carnie snapped the bar over our laps and sent us wheeling upward. I hadn't taken a carnival ride in years. I didn't like the way we swung in our little cup. We were going so much higher than I expected. Normally self-possessed to a fault, I actually did need Dan to hold me. I didn't say anything, but he intuited my feeling. With his arm locked around my waist, I was finally able to look out over the colors of the fair. The ride's vibrations made every buzzing bulb look like flame. It was a timeless, dazzling sight. My hair blew in front of my eyes, and I dropped my shoulders, making myself surrender.

"We have to kiss," Dan said.

A moment later, he asked, "What's happening with your cycle right now?"

He turned his face to my cheek, so close and warm that the intimacy of his question—the first time he had initiated such talk—made me look away.

"I think I'll ovulate in two or three days," I said.

"I was thinking," he said, "maybe we could keep trying. All the way through ovulation, if you want, to improve our chances of making it work."

"Really?"

"We might as well, don't you think?"

An hour later, we hiked out of the enormous fairgrounds and waited for the shuttle bus back to the dirt field where we had parked. As we rode, I peered through the dense huddle of backpacks and shorts, anonymous arms and legs, to find my reflection in the window. I saw my tan shoulder, a swatch of my shamrock-green tank top, my chin, the end of my ponytail. Deeper in the reflection, behind me, sat my beautiful young husband: simple T-shirt, clean profile, dark eyebrows. Watching our bodies and our faces as the bus lurched and leaned, I saw us from the outside: young, naïve, optimistic. I saw us, I realized, in a way our children never would.

A few days later, I plopped into my seat on a flight from Minneapolis to Seattle for a friend's wedding. It was a Friday morning, and I was traveling solo; Dan would fly out that evening after work. I had the whole day to spend with my sister.

The date was September 1, 2006—exactly ten years from the day when Dan and I had met in our college bookstore. It had been the first day of my freshman year, and I stood staring at the sea of bookshelves with an empty basket, looking lost.

"Hello," said a muscular, black-haired boy, crouching in front of the mathematics texts.

"Do you know where the Classics section is?" I asked, looking up from my shopping list. He guessed, pointing toward the back of the store. Later, he would tell me that he hurried to collect the rest of his books so he could stand next to me in the checkout line. As we chatted—lightly with a charge—I glanced into his basket, trying to get an idea of who he was. We didn't have to say much or seize the moment; ours was a small campus, and we knew we'd run into one another again. We did not know, though, that we would become husband and wife, and that exactly a decade from that moment, our cells might create a new life.

All signs indicated that I was ovulating that day. Whenever I paused my reading, I rested my fingers on my abdomen. With the tiniest downward, side-to-center strokes, I willed a healthy egg to pop from my ovary. Each time, I closed my eyes: *Healthy egg, healthy egg . . .*

At lunch, Amanda ordered a glass of wine, and I decided to go with iced tea, just in case. My sister, closer to me than any woman in the world, knew all day that I was sending energy to my ovaries, trying with my mind to choose the egg. She tried with me: "Come on, good egg. Come on," she murmured every so often, as we shared a chicken salad, as we grocery shopped, as we made chocolate mousse for a bridal shower she was throwing, as she hugged me goodbye when I went to pick up Dan.

My sister offered to cradle my secret. She would tell no one about our attempt, our hopes, or our plan. Whether I was becoming pregnant or not, privacy seemed critical now. That evening, Dan and I met a fleet of old college friends in a local bar. Perhaps I should have known better than to draw attention to myself, since a glass of wine wouldn't have hurt. But I ordered ginger ale, thinking that if I kept my body clear of toxins, my chances would be better. I pictured a little lowball glass with ice and a lime; I thought it would look like any old cocktail. So I cringed to see Dan picking his way toward me from the bar, crossing the room with a giant glass of soda, straw and all, held above his head. Anyone who was curious could see that I was choosing not to drink, and it was too easy to guess why.

All night, friends sidled up to me. "You and Dan are next, you know. When's it gonna be?"

I trusted each one of these old, dear friends, but I couldn't stand to reveal anything about our situation. If I said anything, I would want to confide everything. I couldn't simply smile and say, "We're trying," because I couldn't bear the thought of people hovering, even in a well-meaning way, waiting for news that I was pregnant. To them, of course, "pregnant" would mean "expecting." How could I ready myself for the possibility of interrupting a pregnancy while friends and family awaited baby news?

So, I made it sound as far off as I could. "Maybe next year," I said. "Maybe the year after. We'll see." And I smiled, nodding in agreement. "It would be fun, wouldn't it?"

* * *

"Happy birthday," I whispered to Dan as we awoke the next morning in my parents' home. He smiled. Sun streamed through the window, sliding along a moist morning breeze. The air in Seattle always felt like home. In it, we tasted the salty Puget Sound, smelled evergreens and duff, heard the gripes of crows and gulls.

A few hours later, we stood in the middle of a crowd outside Pike Place Market, watching a giant gray macaw dance on a man's shoulder. We each held a sun-warm peach, almost too big to grasp in one hand. We waited for a little pocket to open in the crowd, smiled at each other, then bit in. Juice splattered everywhere. We slurped the amber rivulets that rolled across our palms and down our wrists. A minute later, we each held ruby-red pits. We walked back to the stalls to buy a basket of wild blackberries. Even in Seattle, where blackberries fruited along every highway, they were expensive. The people ahead of us in line made conservative purchases: just enough for two tarts, or maybe a small pie. And no kid fingers dipping in, or there wouldn't be enough. But we grinned and bought a whole pint to gobble on the spot. We slipped out of the shady row of stalls back into the sun, downing the warm berries like popcorn. Fanning our purple-stained fingertips in the salt breeze, we walked back to the car. It was the most perfect breakfast we could imagine: the taste of home. For a moment, we remembered our roots—our identities as creatures from a certain corner of the earth. Distantly, it occurred to me that those perfect fruits might have been our baby's first meal. But I didn't share my thought with Dan. The least I could do for his birthday, I knew, was to give him a break from all my obsessing.

By the end of the wedding weekend, I was exhausted. Too many late nights had me fighting a sore throat. On Sunday afternoon, I went to the guest room in my parents' house to change my shoes—and woke up two hours later when my sister poked her head in. "Are you okay?"

"I'm just exhausted," I said. I grabbed a tissue. During my dead sleep, my sinuses had clogged.

By the time the plane had us back in Minneapolis, all I could do was rest. For two afternoons in a row, instead of working on the writing class I was planning, I slouched in front of the TV. I watched Oprah, local news, national news, even soaps after lunch. My mind seemed to make a washing sound, like slush in a well. By Wednesday, I knew I had to leave the house, or I might sleep for the rest of the century. I decided to head to the copy shop to pick up the reading packets for the class I would soon be teaching. It took me all morning to get showered, dressed, and out to the bus stop. And after I had the packets—two heavy boxes full—I stepped back onto a bus. It didn't take long for me to realize that I had boarded the line headed in the wrong direction; I was on my way into St. Paul, not back through Minneapolis. I slumped over the boxes on the seat next to me, too exhausted to get off the bus. I just kept riding, hoping the driver would let me ride back with him when the route ended. I had no idea where I was going or how long it would take. I was unfamiliar with St. Paul. I had no schedule or route map, and I was overloaded with more than I could carry. My mind was too sluggish to strategize my next move. I was already late for an appointment in Minneapolis, but I couldn't summon the energy to care. I rode on and considered falling asleep. Half an hour passed. My mind feebly rotated through half-baked action plans. Finally, when I saw a safe-looking bus shelter on the opposite side of the street, I pulled the cord and lugged my boxes off the bus. I knew I might have to sit and wait at the bus stop for half an hour or more. But at least I could rest.

"Something's going on," I told Dan at dinner that night. I told him all the guilty little secrets I'd been piling up that week— the TV watching, the incessant napping, my confusion and low resources.

"You're sick," he said, paying so little attention that it surprised me. "You'll be better tomorrow."

He was right, though. By the next day, I felt well enough to go out for a walk. After dinner, we held hands and strolled to the band shell at the lake to hear the summer's last concert. We shared ice cream, hovering in the grass near one family's picnic blanket. None of them were around—probably up dancing—so I cocked my head to read the titles of the children's books fanned over their blanket and chairs.

Dan must have seen my eyes shining with the idea of sitting in the sun reading with my children. "We need to get you pregnant," he said, nudging me.

We walked past the crowd and into the nearby wildlife sanctuary. Cottonwood leaves had begun to turn yellow. They shook, trying to free themselves. The evening sun was warm, but the forest floor seemed cool, sighing in relief as summer's stream of visitors slowed to a trickle. We seemed to be the only people in the woods. I walked just ahead of Dan, as I often did, urging him along with a stride a bit longer than his. But he stopped me with a sudden firm hand on the back of my neck. He turned my head with his hands, so as not to use words. And there in a tiny stream, in the middle of the city, with strains of big band music still reaching us, stood a pretty doe. She spread her front legs and dipped her head to drink. From deeper in the sanctuary, two more deer approached.

I had heard that foxes lived in this tiny strip of wilderness. I had met other walkers who told me that wood ducks nested there, and even beaver could be seen. I knew that deer frequented the sanctuary, but I had never seen one there. I exhaled in appreciation, but it wasn't the animal I felt so thankful for. It was my husband, who knew how to stop me in my tracks, shift my gaze, and make me smile, all without saying a word.

The sanctuary emptied us into the city rose garden, where we wandered among the beds, waving away sunset gnats. I bent to sniff the biggest, brightest blooms we passed. And I noticed something odd. Each one smelled unique. I had grown up in a yard full of my mother's carefully tended roses, yet I had never noticed this before. Dipping my nose into bloom after bloom, I smelled cider, then peaches, then young green fruit, then cinnamon, then baby powder.

"Can you believe this?" I gushed to Dan.

He teased me with a roll of his eyes.

Two weeks after I had spent a sweet Seattle day with my sister, my cold was gone. I had energy again. My brain still made the slushy sounds, though, and I was finding it difficult to dredge up vocabulary. I misspelled when I wrote, rereading one e-mail to find I had used *tu* for the number *two*. My dreams were lively and strange. My period was not yet due, but with the odd sensation of wearing earplugs wherever I went, I felt curious enough to unwrap a pregnancy test. Fumbling more than usual, I caused an error on the stick before I even sat down to pee. The instructions said the test would require half an hour to reset. I used the toilet, guzzled a glass of water, wrapped the stick in tissue, and stuffed it into my purse. We needed groceries.

Picking through produce, wandering the cereal aisle, selecting chicken breasts, I waited for the urge to pee again. When it came, I parked my cart outside the store restroom and locked myself in a stall. It was such a pretty market—they even kept fresh flowers on the bathroom counter. *It wouldn't be a bad place to find out I was pregnant*, I thought. But it didn't matter; NOT PREGNANT, the stick said. With a small shake of my head, I tossed it into the trash. I washed my hands and finished my shopping, convinced the test was wrong.

I had promised Dan I would summon the energy for another weekend adventure. We settled on a day trip to Memphis—short flights there and back, with plenty of time to rent a car and get a feel for the city in a day. So, Saturday morning at sunrise, we made the quick drive to the airport. I surprised myself by actually feeling the energy I had pledged to find. Perhaps I felt a buzz because of the little secret I held: My period still hadn't started. It was only a day late, but even a single day's delay was a significant sign.

It was a sticky day in Tennessee. We combed Memphis by car, trolley, and foot. We sweated as we walked along the Mississippi, cooling down in the air-conditioned café where we ordered barbecue pork and beans. Dan couldn't stop grinning. He loved these crazy junkets—the province, it seemed, of only the rich and the airline-employed—and he kept pulling out the camera to snap souvenir photos.

"Don't move," he said as I stood on a bluff overlooking the river. He seemed to want me in every picture; I felt him appreciating me. But I couldn't focus on myself or my husband. I fixated on the spark I felt in my low abdomen. Every time I smiled for one of Dan's snapshots, I thought, *These are the first pictures of me pregnant.*

The words passed through my mind with conviction, but I didn't entirely believe them. Even when I accidentally belched like a bullfrog on our flight home, I still didn't know for sure what was happening. But the next morning, as we lay in bed on one of the first days to really feel like fall, I took my daily temperature and pulled out my chart to record it.

"Dan, seriously," I said. "I really think I'm pregnant."

"Yeah?" he asked, not even rolling over to look at me. His reservations hadn't gone anywhere; he had only stuffed them. Now, I was calling them up.

"What should we have for breakfast?" he asked, changing the subject so fast that I thought he was kidding.

"Okay, listen," I said, pulling his shoulder so I could see his face. "I know you read the chapters like I asked you to. How many high temperatures in a row indicate a pregnancy?"

"Sixteen," he recited.

"And how many do I have on my chart? Count them."

He did, his finger dutifully marking its way across the page. He tried to keep his voice confident and steady as he counted out loud to sixteen.

"So, what does that tell you?"

"I think it means . . . you're pregnant." He swallowed and buried his head in my side. I heard an alien giggle, a cross between shock and confusion, bundled into an attempt to sound happy.

While Dan showered, I used the last pregnancy test in the box. This time, it took only a second. PREGNANT appeared in the little gray window. I held the stick inside the shower curtain.

"Can you read that?" I asked, tuning to his voice.

"Yes," he said, steadier now.

Later, we walked together to the lake, kicking the first fall leaves. The sun shone with a gleaming Hail Mary force, straining to postpone winter. I loved the feel of the air, the smell of the lake, the sound of squabbling ducks in the water. Dan talked about football, plans for the coming week, goofy places we could fly. Every few minutes, airplanes crossed the cloudlessness overhead. Each time Dan went quiet, I wondered if he was thinking about the pregnancy. But he never brought it up. He gave no sign that the news had registered with him at all.

I, on the other hand, could think of nothing else. I wanted to talk about the pregnancy, to jump for joy, to celebrate. But in truth, we had no idea what lay ahead. By Thanksgiving I would either be three months along or empty again. As Dan watched the airplanes pass, I wondered if he might feel freed—handed a second chance at youth—if we didn't end up continuing the pregnancy.

"I really want to talk about this," I eventually said as we walked. "I'm excited about it, and I want to share it."

"Yeah?" He left an opening for me to talk more. But what I really wanted was to hear him say he was excited, too. As we strolled, he took deep, relaxed breaths and said nothing.

"When do you think this will be real for you?" I asked, trying not to sound angry.

"That's easy," he said, bending to pick up a stick. "When your belly expands."

"But that's after the test!" I lowered my tone and said, "I could go all the way through a termination and never show at all."

He had no response. A new truth settled over me. The next three months were going to be more lonely and painful than either of us had imagined. We would struggle to appreciate one another's positions. For both of us, my existence was now defined by the pregnancy, its tentative nature, and the life changes it could represent. But while I craved a constant listener to help me explore my emotions, my husband needed just the opposite: a partner whose identity was something other than *pregnant*, and a friend who could distract him, supporting his need to pretend nothing had changed—at least not yet.

As the weekend passed, Dan tried to engage me in activities and conversations about anything other than our baby. He invited me out to a new restaurant and, cringing, even offered to spend a whole day shopping with me. My one-track mind was delighted to consider a new menu, mainly because I looked forward to heartfelt words about the pregnancy over our meal. As my husband tried to entice me with ever more exotic travels, I begged off, asking instead for ease: short flights, comfortable beds, impossibly gentle cuisine, not too much walking. As for shopping, I was ready to abandon my old favorite shops; I wanted to see the local maternity boutiques. In between outings, I poked around online, searching for the right combination of baby gear.

"Everything we buy should be nice and lightweight for traveling, right?" I asked Dan, angling for his attention. He barely responded, taking cover in a football broadcast.

After a few days of exchanges like these, it was clear: I was going it alone. *Maybe every pregnant woman does,* I consoled myself, miles from understanding that Dan felt just as isolated.

* * *

"I need to talk about this," I told him again later that week. "I need to talk to someone about it every day. If it can't be you, I have to tell someone else. I want my close friends to know what's going on. I think we should tell some people."

"I'd rather not," he said. "I'd really rather keep this to ourselves."

"Why?"

"If other people know—"

"Then what?"

"Then it feels more real. It feels like it's really happening."

"Well," I snapped, "it is really happening."

Upstairs, behind a closed bedroom door and with my head tucked between Dan's dresser and my closet door, I dialed my sister.

"Where the heck have you been for the past few days?" she said. "You didn't call me back."

"I know."

"Well, what's going on? Did your period come?"

"No," I said, my voice low and overcontrolled.

Excitement rose in her tone. "Did you take a pregnancy test?"

"Yes."

"What did it say?"

"It said I'm pregnant."

"*Oh* my gosh," she said, weirdly guttural. I tried to decipher the emotions that mixed to give her voice a deep, choked sound. Certainly, there was a plunge of adrenaline and fear. A sense of eyes-closed leaping into a deep swimming hole. There was some sadness, too—our shared state of girlhood compromised. And the frustrating inertia at the beginning of a long wait. Stuckness, as we breathed through an overwhelmed silence, unable to let it all go in an embrace.

"How have you been feeling about things?" she asked when she regained her voice. And kept asking, almost every day thereafter. My sister was two years out of college, Catholic, and uncertain about where she stood on certain matters, including whether she even wanted to be tested for HED. She knew all my plans, and it was clear that someday, her own path might look quite different. Still, every morning, when I knew Dan still needed his space, she gave me her ear and carried me with her voice.

paula

I can still hear Mom screaming. "My God! *Oh* my God! They're going to go over!" She kept honking the horn. My dad and brothers were in the U-Haul in front of us. I could see the back of the trailer swerving back and forth across the center line, and they kept teetering over the cliff edge above the river. My dad was practically falling asleep at the wheel while we followed them in the car. Every time my mom screamed I sat up as straight as I could, but I still couldn't see them very well, so I just concentrated on my hangnails, and when my mom wasn't looking I sucked the blood. Then it would be quiet again for a while. It was the Snake River down below us—we were in Idaho—and I thought it looked like mint toothpaste. The rocks seemed chalky and soft. But I knew my brothers and father would die if they went over.

When they climbed into the cab with Dad, my mom told Greg and Curt that their one job was to keep Dad awake. She told them to ask him lots of questions about every little thing they could think of, like different kinds of rocks or tortoises or manufacturing facilities or how tractors run, or math problems, and when you drive an ambulance, how fast can you go, and when do you have to use the siren and lights, or what about his inventions and architecture and when we were born—any of those kinds of things. "But don't say *Junior*," she said. "Remember, your dad is trying to forget."

But I knew my dad. He would just say something like "Your mom said, 'Don't let Daddy take any pills,' didn't she? It's okay, you guys. These pills just make Daddy feel better. See, they're just little and yellow. Your mom doesn't know I'm not feeling very good today. I didn't have a chance to tell her yet." And then he'd be sleeping on the steering wheel.

When we made it down and out of the mountains, my mom said, "Look, Paula! Look at the way the water glitters! That's Lake Washington, and it has floating bridges all the way across. Seattle has quite a shine, wouldn't you say? And all the sailboats!"

When they had the same shift, my mom and dad went to the hospital together, and I would watch Curt after school. But it didn't last long. She came home red-faced one day and yelled at Dad, "Earl, our kids have been so proud of you going to work, you and me both leaving and wearing proper uniforms. And it's not going to last more than five minutes. It's going right down the tubes. I saw you this morning. I saw you drifting through the hospital pharmacy with your long old fingers reaching in there and taking whatever you wanted. Don't you think they know?"

My dad always had that feeling, as if no one had any idea what he was thinking or what he was up to. He thought he was a step ahead of everybody else. When he was a kid, it might have been true. But later it wasn't.

"Well, how long do you think it's going to take them to find out?" my mom yelled.

Pretty soon he was home with us all the time again, on the couch.

"So now what are you going to do with your days?" my mom demanded.

None of us could believe what he said. As if he hadn't learned anything. "Something will come through. I have time. I'm not going to stoop and do something lowly."

He spent all the time sleeping in the living room. It was always the same, in the late afternoons. I'd go in there and say, "Dad, wake up." And then I'd wait.

"Dad, wake up."

"Dad, Dad, Dad, Dad, Dad."

"Can't you get off the couch? Dad?"

"Well, I guess you don't care, but I made some rice and stuff."

A little later he'd start moving around a little. Dinner would be over. Mom would still be at work. And we knew just what was coming.

"Paula! Or Greg? Could one of you guys make me a milkshake?"

He always went on about how good a milkshake sounded. "Oh, yeah yeah yeah, a milkshake would go down just perfect. But I can't really try to get up and make one." He was wobbly all the time.

Mom told us when Dad asked for a milkshake we were to just go in the kitchen and make a little tiny bit. Just one blob, enough to cover the bottom of the cup. She said to use the cups you couldn't see through, and he wouldn't know the difference. We were supposed to put a spoon in it and everything, and give it to him like it was perfectly normal. "Because he'll choke if he's in that state and he tries to swallow too much milkshake," she said. "Just keep an eye on him."

Greg and I would watch from around the doorway and try not to giggle too loud. It was a weird sort of laugh, like we wanted it to be funny, but really it was so strange that it scared us. The way he would look so blissful, scooping and humming over those empty bites with his eyes closed.

I started going over to babysit the little boys next door. Their mom said she'd seen the way I played with her kids around the juniper bushes between our yards, with the blue jays flapping around. She told me how much the little boys liked it when I entertained them and showed them things, so she said she knew I'd do a good job babysitting them. I was eleven. It was my first babysitting besides my brothers, and I started to make a little money. That first night, I got all the hamburgers made for dinner, and I got the two boys to bed, and then it was quiet. I didn't know if their parents were coming home soon or not, so I decided to do a little of my homework. I turned on all the lights in the house so it wouldn't be so dark. But I didn't have a pencil so I started looking around for one. I looked in the kitchen, and then I opened up the drawers in the little desk in the hallway. I saw some stamps that were pretty and a couple postcards and keys and rubber bands. Then I remembered I wanted a pencil, so I got one and went back to the kitchen table.

When I got home my dad said, "Paula, I could see you in there. From the upstairs window. You did a good job babysitting. You made dinner and you cleaned up and put everybody to bed, and I was so proud of you. But I saw you looking around at things that weren't yours. Don't snoop, Paula. Never snoop in other people's business."

But I had to. It somehow fell to me, the job of keeping an eye on my dad. When there was a problem, Mom wanted me to keep my brothers out, to make them stay on the other side of the door no matter what was happening. The first time it got serious, I was just trying to go to the bathroom. I walked in there, and my dad was on the floor by the toilet. His pants were down, and I had never seen him like that. I tried not to look. I tried not to breathe so fast when I picked up the phone and called my mom at the hospital. I was so glad they put her on. "Mom! Dad is on the floor in the bathroom like he fell off the toilet or something. His eyes are closed and everything."

"Is he breathing?"

"Yeah, he's just asleep I think."

She told me I had to help him up. Just to sitting. Then I could leave him there to rest. She said, "Make sure you shut the bathroom door. Don't let your brothers see him like that."

So I went in and closed the door. I looked at him for a second. I felt like he needed a diaper on his little parts. Something for a baby, to cover himself, because he reminded me of a baby the way he was naked on the floor and so confusing to care for. There wasn't very much room by the toilet, so I tried to hook my arms under his arms and twist a little with my waist and pull him up with my back so he could just kind of get back up on the toilet. My dad looked horribly skinny, but he was so heavy. I kept pulling him. I couldn't pull him any harder. His arms just slid away from me. Then I saw there was a needle sticking out of his shoulder.

I thought he was dying. "Mom, he gave himself a shot or something. It's still in him, and I can't get him up. What do I do? What do you want me to do, Mom? You have to come home!"

She told me to just leave him alone and not touch the needle and to keep the bathroom door shut. "He'll wake up later," she said.

That was around the same time when I saw something at school. That morning Gene told everybody to go to the classroom windows at the front side of the school during homeroom, because he was going to do it. Nobody believed him. We had to look across the street to his house, and we would all see if he was telling the truth.

He had spent the whole lunchtime taking his cat's little kittens and burying them in his front yard. He buried them so their little necks came up out of the grass. I could see their tiny heads reaching up like baby birds and mewing. One of them got its little paw out. A boy behind me said he had watched at lunch and that Gene pounded the dirt really hard so those kittens were not getting out of there. I was thinking the kittens seemed really young and little, where their eyes are still blue. And then Gene came around the corner of his house and mowed them. It was one of those pictures I couldn't get out of my head. Things kept coming in and I couldn't get them out.

My dad called me: "Here, Paula? Can you help Daddy for a minute? I'm in the bathroom." I went in there. He was sitting on the edge of the tub with his shirt off. His skin was so white with purple lines. It looked like boysenberry marble fudge.

He said, "Thanks, Baby Doll. Daddy just doesn't feel good. I just feel so sick, and look, my hands are shaking too much, so that's why I need your help. First, just open that bottle right there. You have to push hard—yeah, yeah. Now, can you reach in there and take out one of those pills? Okay, now I'm going to try to hold this vial of water still, and you be really careful and pull the capsule apart—see how it comes apart? Okay, now pour the powder into the water. Oh, good, thank you, Paula."

I didn't ask why or anything. I couldn't even talk. My heart was just pounding. But after I did it, I saw the needle at the end of the syringe. He put the plunger in the top. He didn't even give me a chance to get out of there. It almost sort of seemed like he wanted me to stay in there, so there would be someone to take care of him. I was frozen in my shoes. He took the needle and stabbed it right into the side of his neck. I couldn't breathe.

When I first walked in there, he had been panting and kind of whimpering. But now his breaths were slow. He started to tip back into the tub. I thought I should catch him, but I didn't dare touch him. I was afraid the needle would stick me. He started slumping down, and his eyes were closing. At the last second, he pulled the needle out of his neck and a hundred tiny dots of blood sprayed the wall.

I ran out of there. Then later I remembered to come back and shut the door.

Before that, I never knew what those blood specks were doing all over the bathroom. I thought someone was squeezing pimples or something. I had constantly been wiping them off the faucet handles and the mirror and the wall by the medicine cabinet, and all that time they had been my dad's.

It was Easter soon after that. I was coloring eggs with Curt on newspapers spread over the table. There were all these specks of dye on the headlines, especially red. I couldn't stomach the sight of them. I had to go onto the porch to get some fresh air. To this day, I can't stand to see specks of spaghetti sauce on a stovetop.

That Christmas, he was gone for most of the holiday season. My mom told him, "Earl, you know it won't be like before. They don't do treatments that way anymore. They understand now, and you won't get hurt this time. They're going to help your body get clean inside, and then they'll show you how to stay like that."

He looked at her. She didn't lower her eyes at all. It wasn't like the time with the Montgomerys. It was just her, asking him to do it.

"Here are the papers," she said. "Once you sign I'll drive you straight there and everything can get started. You can be home for Christmas."

And he was. The day he came home, Mom shopped for a big dinner and said we could all celebrate together. She told us he did a good job, and we wouldn't even recognize him. She seemed so proud and happy. She drove to get him, and I got started pounding the chicken and opening the beans. Greg and Curt just kept watching their show and didn't even act excited. I tried to get them to be happy: "Come on, guys, Dad is coming home!" Greg said he didn't want to fall for it. I guess he kind of knew better. I thought maybe I should be more like that. But when our parents came through the door, it felt so good to hear them laughing and see them kissing like that. It made me melt.

In the hall upstairs, Greg said to me, "There's no way this is going to last." But from where I stood, there was no way he could be right. I could hear our parents giggling and whispering down there. Mom missed our dad when he was gone. And now things were the way they were supposed to be.

But of course Greg was right, and it only lasted a few months. He couldn't get a job. He got depressed and miserable again. I was thirteen by then, and I was getting to the point where I kind of felt like I had a life outside of my dad and his behavior. At least a little. School was almost out, and all I could think about was everything we were going to do that summer. Take our skimboards down to Alki Beach and ride across the sand flats. Get the seaweed out of our toes and just soak up the sun.

It was a cold day for June, but me and Rosalie were wearing our bikinis anyway. We always did. We just put on our jackets when the wind picked up. I had my camera, and I asked Curt to take a picture of us girls. My dad was there that day—sometimes he wanted to come down to Alki with us and lay outside, instead of on the couch. I never liked it when he came down. I did like the idea of having my father spend time with us, but not like that. Not the way he was. Curt got ready to take the picture, and Dad said, "Wait, wait—let me get in there," and he huddled in. He put his arms around me and Rosalie, and he smiled softly in the windy sun. When we got back to our towels, I looked over at my dad for a long time. He had all his clothes on—long trousers, long-sleeved shirt. He was so skinny, and he looked cold. I remember thinking he should have been out looking for a job. Anywhere but there with us. Rosalie said, "Glad I had that jacket on for the picture."

"What's that supposed to mean?" I asked.

She said something about how my dad put his arm around us. How he was a creepy old man.

I had never thought of my dad as old. I watched him lying there on his blanket, over by my brothers and their friends. He was basically bald—just a few thin hairs—and he wasn't wearing his hat. Since he had hardly any eyelashes or eyebrows, you could see where his bones bent, and you could see his wrinkles. He did look old.

"He looks as old as my grandpa," said Rosalie. "He even sucks his teeth, see?"

I knew she was right, but I didn't say so. I just said, "He's only thirty-six."

That summer was a particularly good time for observing a certain high school senior practicing football moves in his backyard. "Oh, yummy," I'd say under my breath, and then, "Curt, you want to go play outside with me for a while? I'll just go out and wait for you." Once I went out the side door, which I didn't usually do, but the views were better that way. Mom had said the raspberries were coming along, too, so I wanted to see if I could pick some and peek through the vines at the same time. I walked around the corner, and I practically tripped on my dad. He looked up at me, startled, as if I was a babysitter and he was a kid caught squeezing out all the toothpaste. He swung his head around fast and sucked in his breath. I saw his little plastic glue bottle roll in the dirt.

"Oh my God! I can't believe this! I am so disgusted!" I could really lay into him. "How could you do this? Oh, I can't believe it! I am so, so sick of you!"

I wanted to kick all the sandy soil into his eyes and face. I wanted to knock him down the hill so he rolled into the driveway like an empty pop can. I wanted to shake and shake him. He was so small-looking on the ground there. It seemed like I could pick him up by his paper shoulders and rattle him.

"Oh, Paula, Paula, no, it's not what you think," he said. But it was. By then I knew.

"Dad, what am I supposed to do with you? We've already spent our whole lives loving you more than you deserve. It's hard work! And you can't even love us back and do the right thing. Why can't you love us?"

He held up his two hands like, "Don't hurt me, don't hurt me." As if I could do anything to him.

He started locking himself in the bedroom for the afternoons. For privacy, or to protect us from whatever he was doing. Once I was sitting with Rosalie on the couch watching TV after spending the whole morning at the beach. I spent half of my energy watching the screen and the other half hoping and praying my dad would just stay in his room. *Please please please don't come out here.* I never wanted my friends to even know he was home. But soon enough, he opened up the door, and my heart started pounding because I was still hoping he would walk into the kitchen or somewhere else—just not over to us. *Just go back in there and go to sleep.* But he came right to the couch and said, "Hi, girls!"

Rosalie said, "Hi," politely.

I said, "Dad, what are you doing? Aren't you pretty tired? Aren't you a little under the weather? Don't you think you should go back to bed?"

But he said, "Oh, no no no, I'm feeling very good." Then he walked over to the window and said, "Girls, have you looked out here?"

Rosalie and I looked at each other.

"Come here! Look!" he said. "It's snowing!"

"No it's not, Dad," I said. "It's summer."

But he said, "Yes, it sure is, come on over here and take a look."

So Rosalie and I got up and went over to the window and stood right next to him. We stared out. Everybody was silent. My dad had this little amazed smile on his face. Finally Rosalie kind of laughed a little, like my dad must just be teasing us. So I laughed a little, too. But he kept insisting and watching his imaginary snow without cracking a smile or anything. Rosalie looked at me funny. I just shrugged. I hated that she could see I was just as confused as she was. A kid should be able to understand her own parent. I knew what Rosalie had to be thinking: *Paula Hickman has a totally messed-up dad. A psycho. A druggie.*

When Rosalie went home, I told my dad he had to stay in his room if I ever had a friend over. Which I hardly ever did, because of him. I said he had to swear he would stay behind a locked door. But he wouldn't swear it. Instead he just said, "That's enough out of you." He put a little smile on his face like he adored me.

One day, he tried to cook some chemical in the basement when Mom was at work, and he spilled it all over his lap. It burned right through his pants and skin, all the way to the muscle. He made me so mad with all his accidents and sneaking and hallucinating. He embarrassed me so much. I decided I wasn't going to call him Dad anymore. I would say "my father" if I ever had to talk about him. But he didn't make it easy because he did still try, sometimes. Just when I was sure he would never do anything for us again, he'd decide not to flop down on the couch. He'd say, "What does everybody want for dinner? Want me to make us all some hot dogs?" And in a moment like that I'd just lose myself. I'd walk right over and put my arms around him. He was so skinny. He was barely as big around as me, and personally I could barely get a miniskirt to stay up. I'd give him a huge hug and say into his chest, "I love you, Dad." I couldn't control it.

He wanted Mom to see him doing good things, too. One day, it was like he finally noticed that I'd been going to Sunday school all those years. I guess I started going in Pine Bluffs because I was bored, and then it just became a habit and a social thing. If we didn't live by a church, I would just ask some people at school where there was a good youth group, and later the kids in the group would start to be my friends, like Rosalie. Then it was up to me to keep them, to not let my weird family scare them off.

When Dad finally noticed I was going to church, he wanted all of us kids to get baptized. He kept telling us that he was baptized and this was important. The water would cleanse us through. So he took us to the little church up on Thirty-Fifth, and Pastor Brown poured water on our foreheads. That was fine, but we didn't stay for the cake and punch and all that. Dad thought we should stay, but my brothers didn't want to hang around and jibber-jabber, and neither did I. So we just went home, and Dad told us we had to sit around and wait for Mom to get home from work. He wanted to tell her he did that good thing for us, and he needed to have us sitting there as proof, I guess.

When I started high school, I needed everything to be in its place. I had this pretty little blue scarf I liked to wear around my neck. I had to have it tied exactly right. In the mornings, sometimes it took so long to get it perfect that I didn't even have time for breakfast. But it stayed perfect for the whole day. I would check every time I went to the bathroom between classes. Same with the belt on my coat, same with the way I folded my lunch bag, and same with my pep buttons. In my room I had ten straight pins in a level line on the wall. Greg helped me get them perfect. On the tips of the pins I hung all my pep buttons from school, which I wore on rally days, but usually I just displayed them in my room. They said things like CHIEF SEALTH SALUTE and CLASS OF '72, and there were all the rivalry ones like PLUCK THE EAGLES and SPLIT THE SPARTANS and BAG THE BULLDOGS and BOTTLE RAINIER. I straightened every one of them whenever I ran up to my room and slammed the door to get away from everybody. I was known for my door slamming. My mom said that made the third-floor bedroom perfect for me, even though the walls weren't even finished and the silver paper around the insulation always made weird reflections and scared me.

At night, he smashed into the stairs and crashed along the hallways. I could hear him falling down, and his knees shook the walls when they hit the floor. My pep buttons kept coming down and clanking and rolling all over the floor. I would get up and turn on my lamp and put all the buttons back on their pins perfectly straight like they were supposed to be, and then go back to bed and lay there. Five hundred times a night. *Crash clank clatter roll,* down would go the buttons, and I had to get up and hang them all straight again.

But one time when I heard all the buttons rattle down, I was so mad that I got out of bed and whipped open my door. There he was, crawling on his hands and knees. I just started kicking him and kicking him. I could feel his hip bones and his leg bones with my foot bones. I kept kicking and kicking him down the hall, screaming, "Get away from my room!" Pretty soon my mom came running up the stairs in her nursing uniform. She dropped her keys and went down on the floor next to my dad and yelled at me. "Paula! Stop it! Don't you hurt him! He's sick! He doesn't know!"

That helped me. To see that somehow she still loved him.

The next night, I walked into the kitchen and said, "Mom, Dad, do you need help with dinner or something? What's going on in here?"

They were talking about sending Dad to treatment again, and she'd filled out the top part of the form, but he couldn't make himself sign the bottom.

"Why not?" I asked. I looked at my mom. "Why won't he sign it? Dad, just quit crying and sign the form. Don't you want to get better? Why are you *crying* about it? Mom, what's wrong with him?"

"It hurts him," she said. "He doesn't want to be like this."

"Then what's his problem? *Sign* it, Dad!"

He signed it and walked out of the room. My mom picked up the form and looked at his signature. "Flattened. Like a dog always thinking it's going to get whomped over the head."

"Why are you feeling sorry for him?"

"What is he supposed to do?" she asked me. "Just look at him. His long bones and swollen hands and wheezing chest. His nose is so dry at night it sucks and sticks. Every month he has a cold or a cough or worse. He is in pain. They will take him off his drugs and then what? Should he just bear all of this?"

"Yes," I said. "For us."

earl

The treatment programs didn't leave any more burn marks on my brain; all they did was humiliate me. If humiliation worked, I would have stopped everything a long time ago. The psychiatrist took my history, and I was totally honest. But it didn't matter. They treated me like a regular addict. Like a junkie, like every other person there. They gave me coupons to save for the times I really needed pain medication. I was very careful to read anything I signed, and this place made me swear never to ask a doctor or nurse other than my own psychiatrist for drugs. Or I would be sent home. But what was I supposed to do then, when I still couldn't sleep at 5:00 AM, desperate, my body vibrating and hurting and dead to the touch all at the same time. "You're bleeding. Right through your pajamas," the aide said when I walked onto the ward just before sunrise. My thighs. Those wounds were so deep I never even felt them.

"I can't sleep," I said. "You have to help me."

They hated to see me use my coupons, but when I did, I pleased them in every way. I went to the dance and waved my arms above my head and clapped and smiled and sang. High marks. I finger-painted. Happy nurses. I chatted and asked people

questions about themselves and kept my eyes wide and interested. Satisfied doctors. When I didn't use the coupons, when
I was just me and miserable, they always reported to the next
staffer that I remained asocial. "He only speaks in response to
questions," they'd say in front of my face. "He dressed and came
to the dance last night, but he left right away."

Pages of *The Seattle Times* came through the ward every day.
It was one of the only reasons I came out of my room. There was
my son, on the sports page, jumping, scoring. He looked like me.
They said my will to be a good father was strong enough for me
to overcome my addictions.

paula

My dad was great again, for a little while. As soon as he got out of treatment, he moved us to the house on Webster Street. He was so proud to finally get us into a house he owned again. From the living room windows, we could see the water and the ferryboats way down below. I had my fifteenth birthday in that house. That was my last birthday with our whole family living together.

For a while, he was his old gentle self. Not one little bit of stumbling into the walls or sleeping on the couch during the daytime. That little squeeze bottle didn't seem to come with us to the new house. I snooped around everywhere trying to find it, and it really wasn't there. He kept smiling and hugging us like he hadn't seen us in forever. He said, he couldn't believe how pretty I looked.

But I was scared he was going to fall apart again. I kept fretting about him and watching everything he did, and he could tell how suspicious I was. He said, "Listen, Paula, quit worrying so much about what I'm doing all the time. I might not be wearing a suit, but that doesn't mean I'm not earning money. It's like your mom keeps trying to tell you—I'm not completely healthy these days. Because of that, we're getting Social Security money. And in the meantime I've got an idea or two that may just make you very proud of your papa."

My mom asked him to do just one thing: Get us a second car. The Dart wasn't running, so she wanted him to trade it in and get financing for something that would be reliable enough for me to learn on. But the bank had sent a letter denying them an auto loan. She read it out loud to him. "Earl, it says 'the factors that existed at the time of the loan decline in 1969 preclude the new loan.'"

"What factors?" he asked.

"What do you mean, 'What factors?' Don't act like you haven't been here. Maybe a bankruptcy? Maybe you didn't pay our taxes for four years running? Maybe you, just sitting around all the time on disability even though you could get up and work if you weren't such a wimp about it? Maybe the same factors that make it so half the time I can't cash my paycheck because every wage I make is garnished? You are making it impossible for us to live, Earl," she said. "To just *live*."

Then came the afternoon when we heard it again, from the living room: "Paula? Are you home? Or Greg? Can somebody fix milkshakes for everybody?"

My mom found his drugs and took them from his hiding places and put them into other hiding places.

"Do you kids know where your mom put my medicine?" he would ask us. It was one of the only things that would make him really mad. "She's a witch! A sick, evil witch! How can she not understand? She's a medical woman. Where did she put everything? Greg? Paula! You better not be hiding anything from me, your father. Do you hear me? Answer me!"

Once he was so mad he kicked a hole in their bedroom closet. That was as violent as I ever saw him.

He yelled as loud as he could, which wasn't really very loud.

"Paula! Call your mom and tell her I said I need to know right now what she did with all of my medicine. Call her!"

To get around her, my dad kept using this pharmacy, Mike's, which had a delivery service. Mike's daughter went to school with me, and I knew her. Mike would come to our house to deliver all these drugs and see my dad like that, and it was just another way word got out that my family was a mess. I couldn't stand to hear the doorbell ringing, and my dad clattering over there to answer it, so excited like it was going to be a big bag of birthday presents or something. Then he'd go, "Paula! Or Greg! Quick! I need a little change for the tip." He just made me jumpy.

Once I found my mom's recipe for pistachio cake and I made it for myself. It was spring and I was sitting out on the front porch. Things were starting to bloom. It was warm enough for a short-sleeved sweater. I was waiting for my mom to get home and take me for my driving test. I saw the mailman starting to come up the hill. He was gray-haired and he smiled whenever he saw us. But I never wanted to see anybody, especially not at my house, where my dad was always drifting around the window-panes and hanging in the doorways. So I started to go back inside, but the mailman got up the steps too fast and he was right there smiling at me with big wet eyes. He handed me the mail, and I turned around again to go inside, since Mom said to get the mail and hide it as fast as we could, stick it under the couch cushions if we had to, and just not to forget where we put it.

But the mailman didn't go. He was still standing there when I started to shut the door. He said, "I'm really sorry about your dad."

"Oh yeah, thanks," I said. I wasn't sure what he meant.

Then he asked, "Is it cancer?"

I was so embarrassed.

* * *

"You tell me. How can we have you in the house?" Mom said to Dad when she took out the restraining order. "Do I really have to explain? We have to keep you out of here so we can just get by. You take everybody's money you can find. You steal my checks. You hover by the porch waiting for the mail. You think you are a loving father. What kind of father does things like that? How am I supposed to feed the kids and make the house payments?"

She said, "Paula, Greg, Curt, you kids have to call me if you see your dad here at the house, and I'll call the police. Or you can just call the police yourselves."

She and my dad both went out the door—I don't know where she was going to take him. Greg said, "Like we're gonna call the police on our dad."

Curt said, "Yeah."

"Okay," I asked them later, after he came back for a few hours that afternoon, "so how are we supposed to explain to mom where the mail went, and all his toiletries and medicine and the portable TV? We should have called the police. I know he's our dad, but he only causes trouble, in case you haven't noticed."

He was in the hospital for a while right around then. He kept having these nose jobs, to try to clear his breathing, and I think to make his nose look better to him. This time the surgery site got infected, and the infection went into his eyes. He was probably miserable, but we were all relieved to have a break from his hanging around every day. Mom said we could go visit him at the hospital if we wanted, but she said, "Lord knows I'm not going over there. What a relief from all that pestering."

When he was well enough, he kept coming back. I have no idea where he went otherwise. He didn't have anybody else. "What do you expect me to do?" he said to my mom.

Later the divorce papers came. For once, there was a piece of mail he wouldn't touch. My mom got home from work and saw my dad and the envelope sitting there. "If you won't open it, then I will," she told him. "Are you listening?"

He went down the hall. He closed the bathroom door behind him.

She put her mouth up to the door. "Stop slamming around," she said. "'Dear Mr. Hickman, This is to notify you of the trial which has been set for January 15, 1971.' Earl, I know you heard that."

earl

I found a bed at the YMCA. I signed everything for the three-day trial period required before I could apply for the weekly rate. Their rules were written for other men. Not me. They underlined in the application *Women and girls are not permitted on the YMCA residence floors or in the rooms at any time.* That was all I could think about when I pushed the application across the counter. Women and girls. My wife, who was just a girl when I met her, and then the daughter we had, a girl, a baby doll, and how she was a little girl in little girl dresses and little girl shoes, and my wife who was a woman then, with her perfect-fitting blouses and long coats. She always laughed in Broomfield, when she had the lawn chairs out and the sun coming down on her, and my little girl running with the boys. Once, I could hold my daughter in one hand. But now she was tall and slender and pretty and smart. Women and girls not allowed. It was the greatest affront. These women and girls, these particular two, belonged anywhere and everywhere in my universe.

None of the young men there were like me. None of them had accomplishments and families. All they wanted to do was play ping-pong and drink bottles of beer and waste their money on magazines and candy. None of them had owned homes and businesses and real estate. None of them had grown up already, a long time ago.

The radiators clanked and seethed each night. I could not control the temperature of my room. It was too hot to sleep. I just lay there, seeing all the things I had once possessed. But I busied myself. I would recover everything, and more. I didn't play games or watch TV. I tackled the legal matters that barred me from my home and family.

To do: Send letter to Judge, Times, Post-Intelligencer *(all news media).*

RE: Decree of Divorce
Your Honor:
The Injured in this case deserves more than an affidavit. Eighteen years of marriage on two pages of legal paper? My wife has only one contention: the habitual use (however necessary) and financial consequence of my health requirements. I am not the scum previously depicted to you. You have all the bad factors or alleged misdemeanors, but my adult life has not been completely a scourge to mankind. To wit:
• Patents taken
• Sizeable loans given, to help others
Esta is overworked, pressured by outsiders to take this action against me. This is entirely prompted by slanted affidavits from a jealous attorney; my wife is an attractive woman.

By Tuesday: Prepare Brief for Judge's study. Include pictures.

Parent-child interaction: steady and ongoing. Unsuitable home conditions when I am absent. Kids' report cards to demonstrate my involvement. In this system of jurisprudence, quite obviously I have been adjudged guilty unless I can prove I am not a bad influence in the family home.

I can only pray, Sir, that you can, or will, wade through this, and it may spark enough interest to bring about some correction of erroneous impressions. What has happened to the role of the court to mediate or attempt amicable reconciliation? She has attended marriage and family counseling by herself—no contact ever has been made by these counselors to myself. Or to the most injured: the children. How can a man sit in judgment and objectively render a decision when he has not met either of us?

This letter will just be glanced at. The adage "ignorance of the law is no excuse" will enter into play. However, I wish to provide the following for informational purposes: I realize I am to be "out" of the house, but how could anyone remove himself from the one he loves, even if it were financially possible? (I am currently earning $134/month from Social Security. Could you, your Honor, live on this amount?)

I still consider my marriage vows sacred. Parents are a two-headed figure. No person can say I have not loved with all my heart the siblings from this union (which, by the way, was her idea, not mine. She had full knowledge of my habits, shortcomings, health. She still wanted to marry me.) The moral fiber of these kids has, for the most part, been imparted by me. And yes, a subpoena to substantiate this rather braggadocious claim can be obtained.

How delightful things could and should be. She does not realize it, but she does love me.

I was a wonderful person.

Sincerely,
Earl L. Hickman

I could not make them understand. The cards were stacked against me. I was left only with accountings to make. Household goods and furnishings were turned over to Esta. I would be without a car for the first time since I started driving. Each of us was to take our own clothing and jewelry. The rings, etched—did they carry any meaning at all anymore? I had to ask myself then, as I do now, can such failure be lightly brushed aside?

Account of losses:

Wife.

Three children.

Several nice homes and business concerns.
Hair, dentures, body fat, suitable clothing.

Smooth-functioning pharmaceutical drugs—not raw
miscellaneous from the street like this, giving me to
shudders and jerking, my legs collapsing under me,
deliverance to the elevator floor.

Body responsive to oral administration of treatments,
before injections became necessary for similar effect.

Blue pens and a desk and a lamp and children breathing
by my knees. My wife straightening the house after the
day, passing my doorway in her nightgown, silent, soft.

For each irredeemable loss, I dissolved one measure into the syringe. The overdose was purposeful, but I didn't want so terribly to die. I wanted to see my family, and to be delivered from pain. YMCA staff found me in the doorway of my room, and called an ambulance. Paula came to the hospital. But instead of smothering me with kisses, saying thank God I was alive, she said, "Dad, I'm sick of this. How can you not value yourself? I know it's hard, but you have to try to do the right thing."

Dan and I had been planning to fly to California in September for a wine-tasting weekend with two other couples. Eager to see our old college friends, we decided the pregnancy should be no reason to stay home. As the six of us cruised from one winery to the next, I invoked my junior-high acting skills, taking wine into my mouth, tasting, sometimes swallowing, and sometimes spitting. Other times, I just touched the wine to my lips as I had been taught to do when taking communion at church. Even though nothing tasted right, the charade was working—even on my husband. As I worked my way down one counter, Dan hovered with his whole body pressed against mine. "You're not swallowing that, are you?" he asked. I assured him. Later, close to my ear, he whispered again, "How much is going down? Are you being careful?"

Instead of being annoyed by his worry, I appreciated it. His concern was one of the few small ways in which he had acknowledged the tiny presence inside of me. It had been only a week since I'd stuck my positive pregnancy test into Dan's shower. It still seemed generally best not to discuss it.

I wanted our good friends to help talk us through our time

of limbo. Even though it would be unusual among our friends to reveal a pregnancy before the twelfth week, Dan guarded our privacy to the extreme. The six of us sat crammed in a minArt for hours during our excursion, and Dan volunteered the two of us for the far backseat. When I kept falling asleep—an escape from the queasiness—Dan teased me more than anyone else. Still an hour's drive from dinner, I finally felt so protein starved that I demanded a stop and hurried into a Starbucks to order a drink. Back in the car, where everyone thought I needed a strong coffee to correct my mood, only I knew that inside my cup was ice-cold milk. Dan gave no hint that he understood. I didn't know if this was an acting job, like my phony wine tasting, or whether it was simply denial.

The next morning, Dan awoke before I did and wandered into our friends' kitchen to chat and help with breakfast. In my half hour in bed alone, fresh from sleep, my mind careened into a place of fear. What if the news wasn't good? For a moment, viscerally, I felt the deep sadness of our possible loss. The sloshing sound in my head amplified as my thoughts whirled out of control. It was as if I had awakened into the crashing of oceans, the squealing of construction, the shrieking of brakes, and the pounding of drums all at once. I breathed faster, trying to find a way to stop the whiplash between fear and hope. *Quiet, quiet, quiet,* I begged. But my thoughts were too many and too huge. I couldn't hush them. They needed out.

Dan came to see if I was awake, only to find me sobbing into the pillow.

"What's the matter, Kiddo?" he asked, shutting the door and crawling in with me. "You tell me. What?"

"I'm just so sad and confused," I said. "I need someone to talk to—*seriously* talk to. Will our insurance cover a therapist? I need a therapist."

He said nothing, stroking his big hand over my hair as I cried, keeping his breath against my neck. "I'll find out," he said. "But for now, why don't you just tell me?"

"I just don't know how to feel. It doesn't seem right to be happy all the time. I can't just pretend it's all going to be fine, because I'll be too devastated if we get bad news. But I can't go around being sad all the time, either. It's no good for me or the baby or you. There's so much going on, and I can't figure out how to hold everything at once. I just think it might help if I had someone saying, 'You just have to make it through one more week, until our next meeting.' I need mile markers in all this mixed-up waiting. So I can take it a little at a time."

He waited to see if I would say more.

"It's the mornings," I said. "The mornings and the alone times are so hard."

"What's helped you through the mornings so far?" he asked.

"Just being busy. Distracted."

"Well," he said, "there you go. You can come out of the bedroom and hang out now. When we get home on Sunday, we can really make sure you have lots to keep you busy. You have tons of writing to do, and planning for classes, and maybe you'll want to do some projects around the house." He brushed away some of my tears. I didn't take to the idea of work, but I did picture watching sports, going to the movies, stepping out to a coffee shop every day.

"But at the same time," I said, "I don't think it's right to ignore what's going on. This was part of the deal. I think it's important to feel the pain of this. If I pretend it's not happening, I could be haunted for the rest of my life by the pregnancy I didn't stop to notice before it was gone. I have to stay awake to the possibilities for this baby. It just hurts." I let loose another wave, feeling the pillow soak beneath my temple.

Dan held me until I could speak again.

I took a breath. "This is the hardest thing I've ever done."

I stopped, hearing the words I had put into the air. I needed a moment to examine them and to understand that they were true. "If it doesn't work out," I said, "I don't know if I will ever have the strength to do this again."

He squeezed me even closer. "We can find a therapist. We can do whatever you need."

His closeness was the thing I needed most, but he was bearing his own burden and couldn't carry all of mine as well. So, after I dressed, I waved Dan back into the bedroom.

"Dan, I need to confide in a couple of my girlfriends. After that, if I still feel like I need a therapist, then I'll look for one."

"Good," he said, hugging me one more time. "You can do anything you need, okay? Now come on. Waffles are ready."

During my September walks around Lake Harriet, I tried to open my imagination and my heart to many possible outcomes. I could carry no expectations for the pregnancy. I even had to keep expectations at bay for something as simple as the schedule along which its early events would unfold. I had six weeks to wait until our CVS test at the end of October, and an additional two or three weeks to wait for results. The test date—the day before Halloween—was the single fixed milepost in my journey. Dan and I both clung to the hope that we would have our answer before Thanksgiving—well enough in advance to go through with a termination procedure before the long holiday weekend. I couldn't imagine learning bad news just before Thanksgiving and then needing to wait four or five days for the next step. And it seemed like it would be nearly as awful to wait through the holiday weekend without any word at all.

Alongside the worst-case scenarios, I indulged in sweet fantasies. I pictured announcing a healthy pregnancy to our families over tables laden with turkey and dressing. Speed-walking with my eyes full of the round lake and its skirt of shimmying trees, I painted my dearest hopes in every detail: the sweater I would be wearing, the aroma of the meal, the delighted expressions on our mothers' faces. I walked even faster, as if trying to outrun my fantasies, knowing I was only ratcheting my hopes higher and higher with every quick step.

But even though I slipped daily into my Thanksgiving reverie, Dan and I decided early that we would not travel to Seattle for the holiday, no matter what news we had—or didn't have.

"Flights to Europe will be wide open," he grinned. "Where should we go? You choose."

Even though I had been contrary about traveling too much during the first trimester, I agreed that we should plan to leave the country over Thanksgiving, whether we had good news or no news. Bad news would mean we would probably be home alone together, resting and recovering.

It was easy to get caught up in the minutiae of the many possibilities ahead. But one morning, kicking through yellow leaves on my way back from the lake, I remembered myself. I remembered the relationship I had shared for a decade with Dan, and the houses we had lived in, and the routines we moved through. I realized that losing the baby would not be the same as losing myself. *We would still have us*, I thought. I put a question to myself: Would I trade Dan, or my friendship with him, for news of a healthy baby right now? Certainly not. Even if the pregnancy was a quiet topic, we still loved waking up side by side. Each evening before dinner, my ears tuned to the street, listening for his car. Our companionship was my simplest, sweetest pleasure—something I would never trade away. And I realized with a great wave of comfort that I would never have to make such a choice. Healthy baby or not, we would still have ourselves and our marriage—the things I cherished most in the world. In that sense, our gamble could not lose.

My daily walk seemed to save my mind. Though I flung myself through a gauntlet of scenarios as I circled the lake, I somehow managed to return to my front door each day feeling mostly whole.

* * *

Through open windows, early in the morning on the last day of September, the yard smelled lightly toasted. It would be a warm weekend across Minnesota, and Dan and I had decided to take off—but not to fly—for the weekend. We wanted to feel more deserving of the title "Minnesotan," and we knew we had lots of exploring to do. We didn't have enough vacation to strap the canoe onto the car for a full excursion to the Boundary Waters, but we still wanted to head north for a couple of days. By lunchtime, we were barreling toward Duluth, with the windows cracked open and mellow music playing. Leaving my flip-flops on the floor, I propped my feet on the dash. I took mouthfuls of fresh air from the window, trying to keep nausea at bay. As we drove to a higher latitude, we watched the trees change color in succession, like a time-lapse movie of autumn's progress. Reds simmered from cherry to rust, oranges flared from fire to peach, and finally, golds dimmed from sun to ore.

I felt stirred by the rays and color, by the ocean of blue sky. Everything around me called for celebration. Optimism bowled over my sense of caution.

"If we knew we were having this baby," I said to Dan, "we'd be trying to think of names right now."

He glanced over, sunglasses shielding his eyes.

I pressed. "Do you think we can do it anyway?"

"No way," he said. "Not a good idea."

I turned my eyes back to the windshield and the battalions of bright trees. I knew he was right. Music filled our silence as we rode on.

Later, when the tent stood taut and firewood lay in a neat stack beside the pit, we grabbed jackets and struck off into the brush. Giddy with the slow-dying spirit of summer, we bushwhacked our way up a brambly hill. Dan always aimed to get high enough to find a view—a penchant ingrained from his Washington State childhood. At the top of the bluff, though, all we could see were yellow cottonwood leaves. So we stomped and slid back down, following the sound of water to the bank of the Baptism River. Tucked into a low, coppery canyon, we rock-hopped across the shallow current as late-day sun washed the trees, rocks, and water in the antique gold particular to a northern fall. I felt happy to be out in the fresh air, to find my legs springy and strong as we leaped over little rapids. With tamaracks and poplars soaring overhead and the bigness of the sky and earth sandwiching me between, I felt steadied. My mind quieted down. I was with Dan, the two of us soon to be swaddled in our sleeping bags and tiny blue tent, with all the basic necessities tucked into our little Civic.

For the rest of the afternoon, except for a few bouts of nausea when neighboring campers filled the air with exhaust from generators and truck engines, I was able to shuffle thoughts of my pregnancy to a safe place in the back of my mind. I didn't go so far as to forget I was pregnant, but I did let thoughts of the baby recede. We ate our usual sausage-and-tomato sandwiches and, when darkness fell with a sky full of clear silver stars, we sat by Dan's fire, warming our shins as closely as we dared. The air temperature fell below freezing, but I couldn't have been more comfortable snuggled into a down cocoon with Dan. My body settled toward the earth, heavy and content.

We awoke to the feuding of squirrels in a pine tree above the tent. The day was crystalline. We packed up to drive still farther north. Pregnancy still rested just out of sight. We found lunch in Ely, an outfitters' town leading into the Boundary Waters. My queasy stomach gurgled, but a persistent smile hung on my face.

In the thinning woods, we spotted gray jays, ravens, and spruce grouse as we cruised toward a state park. I wore just a T-shirt, knowing this might be the last day of the year when the sun could warm me through. Pausing to take pictures straight up into the candy-dazzle canopy, we hiked around a tiny, forested lake, hidden in a deep pothole. Later, coming to the edge of a larger lake, we sat down to rest on the bank, finding smooth seats on the soil between tree roots and grass hummocks. I untied my shoes and flicked my socks up the bank, dunking my feet into the refreshing cold. Dan looked surprised, but then he did the same. We slid the bottoms of our feet back and forth over mossy green rocks. A bald eagle wheeled above the water, her head and tail a clean, crisp white that blazed against the vivid blue sky. I plucked a piece of grass and tucked it between my thumbs, blowing hard to whistle a ragged squawk across the water.

"How do you do that?" Dan asked.

I positioned his fingers. Soon the two of us were bugling squeaks and wails across the blue water. Around a wooded peninsula drifted a boatful of hunters with the motor cut. Maybe they thought we were mating elk. Plainly visible in our bright clothes, we laughed. Then we closed our eyes and tipped back, letting the warmth soak us.

I drove much of the way home to Minneapolis that evening. Holding the wheel helped me keep from getting sick. As Dan slept, I began passing billboards in a series along the highway back to the Twin Cities. Each billboard featured a bouncing baby, several months old, bright and expressive.

WHAT! I COULD SMILE BEFORE I WAS BORN, one stated, rather inscrutably.

HELLO WORLD! said another. MY HEART WAS BEATING 18 DAYS FROM CONCEPTION.

Even though I knew doctrine when I saw it, the signs were like slaps in the face—invasions of the quiet peace I had managed to cultivate over the weekend. I wondered who believed that women really needed to be reminded that the choice to end a pregnancy is a choice against a life of some kind. I knew I might one day choose against seeing my son's smiles. Against pressing my ear to his chest and hearing his heart thumping like a tight little drum.

Abortions were legal in Minnesota up to twenty-two weeks' gestation, when a fetus would have fingerprints and hair, suck his thumb, and hear sounds from his mother, but would not be able to survive outside the womb—and certainly wouldn't wear size-three diapers or grin with ad-perfect dimples. Against my better judgment, I had been dipping into mainstream books to read about the progress of my pregnancy. Like the billboards, each book eagerly addressed embryonic and fetal development, giving me, week by week, little human characteristics to mourn if we chose to say goodbye to our pregnancy. An abortion following CVS would most likely take place at about fourteen weeks, when our four-inch, translucent-skinned fetus might begin to coordinate the movements of his arms and legs.

As the colossal spokesbabies flashed by, I realized that I wanted a book to reassure me of the things my six-week-old embryo *couldn't* yet do. I wanted to read a single paragraph that took pains to remind me how far from consciousness, from human behavior, my gestating fetus was: *Your baby is one-and-a-half years from being able to interpret simple spoken sentences, and at least two years from speaking phrases on his own. Your baby is at least two years from recognizing himself as a conscious being, and three years from understanding that other people are separate individuals. In five years, he may have the capacity to read written language. He is at least eighteen years from distinguishing information from propaganda.*

But instead, the authors of some popular pregnancy guides actually identified which circumstances might justify an abortion. "If testing suggests a defect that will be fatal or extremely disabling," one said, "many parents opt to terminate the pregnancy."

These passages always caused me to call into question my reasoning. HED wasn't directly life-threatening. Our affected son would be unlikely to die as a child. And I didn't know what "extremely disabling" meant, but I suspected that the authors of the book would not characterize HED that way. Neither would I. Still, reexamining the plans we had made, I didn't feel my path was wrong.

Dan slept in the passenger seat with his head tipped back and his jaw gently open. As highway lights streamed by, anger bubbled inside me. I felt angry that I couldn't shout to the world about what we were going through. I felt alone. I wanted to make friends in Minneapolis—particularly with a group of spunky neighbor gals—but to me, investing in friendship meant sharing, and I had no idea what those women would say if I revealed my tentative pregnancy. Considering the presumptive pregnancy-guide authors and the few people I had told about HED, I had learned that some people would hear only a few words about a disorder before announcing what should be done. Too many times, in trying to describe the complexity of HED to someone, I could tell they were thinking, *That doesn't sound so bad.*

I gave myself a moment to feel disgusted with people's tendency to array health problems along a worseness spectrum: Some are bad, some are terrible, some are "extreme." Conclusions came so quickly to people who had no experience with a disorder in their bloodline. But at the same time, I knew how natural it was to try to approach another person's genetic quandary with logic alone—or with anecdotal experience. I even had my own tidy hierarchy of disease. Deep down, I knew it would be easier for me to consider an abortion if the baby tested positive for a major disorder. Why would I agonize over the choice for a baby with HED more than I would for a baby affected by another disorder? Perhaps because HED felt like family, and a different condition seemed more like a stranger to me. I felt that I knew the little guy with HED. He was familiar to me, a family member I had already met. He had appeared in many of my dreams. In one of his recent visits, my mother walked down a staircase to show me the tiny boy she had adopted, curled and sleeping sweetly in a shoebox. Because of his disorder, his parents had given him away. I looked into the box and immediately began weeping. I felt so sorry for his mother and father. They would miss his beautiful life.

My frustration grew as more billboards passed and the city lights drew closer. I felt angry that my society had made a taboo subject of one of the most important journeys of my life. An abortion—a story that would belong to me, shape me, become a part of me—would henceforth divide people into those who could handle a relationship with me and those who couldn't. It seemed I had two choices: I could live as if I had a terrible secret, or I could live marked. Driving into Minneapolis, I decided I would call my friend Eula in Chicago the next morning to tell her what was happening. I took deep breaths and tucked away my fury.

Just as I had hoped, Eula heard me out. She helped me further my thinking, describing a woman's rights in words I hadn't thought of: "A pregnancy falls within the mother's domain, and no one else's," she said. "Not the public domain, not the church's, and not the state's."

Now that I was carrying a baby, I literally felt what Eula meant by "a mother's domain." I had a moment of physical sickness just thinking about the idea that anyone else might try to claim authority over my pregnancy. Imagining such a thing was one of the most confining, frightening feelings I had known as a woman who had grown up carefree and safe in a nation of so many freedoms. It was the feeling of persecution. *Someone might as well steal my hands and face,* I thought, *and call them their own.*

"But I still feel so guilt-ridden," I told her, "to consider ending a little life just because it is imperfect. This baby would live, and he would probably have a good life. I just can't know. But I'm doing this for the baby," I reminded myself out loud, "not for Dan and me."

Eula let my words hang in the air. Then she said, "Why don't you feel you deserve to have the child you want?"

I was struck. Her words touched the thinking that seemed most dangerous to me, most immoral. Could it possibly be all right, in my America or in some other life in some other place, for parents to want healthy children for their own peace of mind? I thought of my ancestors who, like millions of modern people around the globe, needed plenty of healthy children with strong backs to ensure the family's survival—and with any luck, prosperity. Dan and I had no plans to rely on our children for a livelihood; we wanted children just for the joy of it, just for the journey. Even though we knew a baby without HED would save us tens of thousands of dollars in medical and dental bills, our choice to become pregnant, and our desire for a healthy child, could not be rationalized as economic necessity. It was closer to emotional luxury. Did our quiet wish for a healthy baby mean we had entered the realm of hubris? Had we been swept into the mythical promise of the American Dream, not unlike my grandfather Earl with his ambitions?

In our paradoxical nation, where Puritanical humility was expected to temper every accomplishment, it seemed wrong to want to enact a plan for the best. But thanks to Eula's question, I saw folded deep in my heart a tiny possibility. *Maybe*, I thought, *I should want a healthy baby for myself, and for Dan, and for our marriage and future. It might be noble to shoulder a burden, but it is also good to forestall harm and strive for plenty.*

I kept the thought to myself, holding close its kind whisper of acknowledgement that this was, after all, about me, too. I felt a glimmer of self-love—something I had not allowed before. It marked the beginning of a turning for me, in which I realized I did not have to make myself everybody's victim. If I really believed these choices were rightly mine, then I needed to live like it. I had to stop walking out the door each day expecting to be smacked by another billboard, another injustice. If I allowed it, they would just keep coming.

But my transformation was slow. I still read pregnancy books like an addict, inflicting self-abuse. I couldn't pull my mind away from the details about how much bigger and more vital our baby was becoming. Perhaps this was part of staring our choice in the face. I swung between a resolve to hold at arm's length the blooming reality of our baby's body and the desire to revel in the realness of it, in which I pretended that I knew our baby was healthy and preparing for an appearance the following spring.

"I'm due at the end of May," I told my sister over the phone. "It's the strangest thing to look into my future just seven months and see such different possibilities." I knew I could be hugely pregnant, fixing up a nursery. Or I could be traveling long and hard with Dan, trying to fill an empty womb with sights and sounds and foods from far away. I could become a sudden workaholic, feeding the bank account as a feeble gesture toward the imaginary children of our future.

"You know," my sister said slowly, "you've started the journey toward having a baby, and it's really not going to be over until someone is born. The way I see it, you're going to be pregnant until that child arrives, whether that's eight months from now, or twelve, or twenty-four. This might not be the baby we hold. But you're on your way."

She was right. I felt as if I had jumped into a lake and started swimming, not knowing when I would reach the opposite shore, or even how far it was, but somehow knowing I would make it eventually. The conditions of the lake itself would determine the events of my swim—not my physical strength or mental resolve. I had been thinking of my pregnancy as three months long at minimum, about ten at the max. But Amanda helped me stretch my idea of pregnancy to include another sense of the word: meaningfulness in waiting.

I felt better with the idea that my swim could be all one long, blind backstroke to a distant shore, instead of several dog paddles from the sand to the dock and back. I liked water, but swimming to actually get somewhere had always been exhausting and difficult for me. Holding my pregnancy—the figurative one and the physical one—felt no different. Yet in my dreams, I had been swimming almost every night. I swam through floods, under ice, through choppy shipping canals, and across the bows of ocean liners. I was never afraid. I always knew I would make it. Sometimes I rescued other people who believed they would drown.

I was bursting to talk to my mother. She was an avid dreamer who would relish helping me explore my nighttime swims. But it wasn't just for the pregnancy news or the dreams that I wanted to call her, go to her. I wanted more—or, really, less. I just wanted to be close to her. I walked the lake, shoulders slumped, wishing that she would appear around the next bend, waiting with a hug for me, a rub for my hair. I didn't need words, but I wanted the physical comfort that only my mother could give me. She knew how to soften me: how to gentle my eyes and soothe my straining limbs.

In certain moments, I felt desperate to tell my mother everything and to have her with me as the date of the genetic test drew nearer. But a phone call to Seattle wasn't going to give me the connection that I wanted. And I was tired of words. I knew if I told my mom about the pregnancy and our plan, it would rend her heart. It would pry open years of her own questioning, leaving her with a daunting emotional project. She would need to seek her friends' ears, to spill her secret sadness. At the time, I didn't have room in my head or heart for the guilt I would feel if my pregnancy became anyone else's burden. Someday I would be ready to share, but not now. Not halfway through week seven, when my lungs burned from swimming and my baby's heart had just bloomed into four perfect chambers.

paula

After the divorce, he really wasn't supposed to be coming around. Still, he was there again on my seventeenth birthday. I didn't want him near me. He was starting to smell. I didn't know why he had that smell. He kept pushing his way into all the pictures as though he wanted to make sure we went down as one happy family. He put his arm around me and smiled for the camera as if he was the one who made the cake and lit the candles and cooked my favorite ravioli for dinner, and not just the guy who showed up because he made a good guess about what time there'd be food on the table.

He had this weird new habit with potato chips. He would ask for them as soon as he got to the house—"Hey, do you guys have any potato chips?" Then he'd sit there with a TV tray stacking the chips, and the stack would get really tall. I don't remember him ever getting around to eating the chips—just stacking them. The tray wasn't very stable and it was kind of amazing, but I couldn't laugh about it the way Greg and Curt did. I just sat there thinking, "Why the hell does he need to do that?"

He was in and out of the hospital. Sometimes I wondered if he felt better in the hospital than he did anywhere else. He had a phone and company and regular meals, and the doctors would just keep him on pain medication because of his addictions— they didn't try to get him off drugs, but they did make sure he was taking safe things. Those chemical burns never healed. He put needles into them and they kept ulcerating and getting infected. He'd bleed through his pants. Sometimes the wounds festered all the way down to the bone.

By the time I was a senior in high school, I pretty much avoided him. I started riding my bike to Dr. Johnson's office after school for my first job. I was a bookkeeper and a front desk recep- tionist. I mainly filed things, but I was trained to answer the phone. Dr. Johnson was always so tan and rosy-cheeked. He was wholesome-looking, and he wore that white coat over his suit, and he had a deep voice. He was gentle with his patients and tall, and he listened to them even when they were just chatting on the way out. He was restrained. He let people be. He encouraged me. "Good, good, Paula, thanks for being so efficient with that." I was quick with everything he asked, and when he couldn't think of anything else for me to do, then he'd say, "Well, Paula, have a gorgeous ride home. See you tomorrow afternoon." His house was across the street from the beach, and when I went tanning on hot days, I put my towel in the sand directly in front of his house. It made me feel safe.

Then one day I was straightening some patient files for him, and I saw it, right in my lap on top of the pile: HICKMAN, EARL L. He had come in for prescriptions, just short visits for refills for pain, for depression, for anxiety, for severe insomnia. The next time I saw Dr. Johnson come down the hall, I wanted to die. Now he knew. Everyone always knew.

At home I was snooping around in some things my dad left on the table. He and my mom were fighting in the bedroom, about money I'm sure, and the fact that it was against the law for him to be in the house. Then in his pile of newspapers and notes and his wallet and everything, I found a prescription pad. Dr. Johnson's prescription pad. Stolen. I was furious. I stomped into the bedroom waving the pad. "Dad! Stay out of my life! Can't you not be in every part of my life?"

My mom said, "Well, Earl, do you want to tell her what else?"

He didn't say anything.

She said, "Paula, you should know that this idiot also has been going to the fathers of your friends from church and your friends from school, so you better not tell your dad your friends' names anymore. The second you tell him a name, he's on their doorstep, telling their father about your inspiring friendship and our family's epic struggle and asking to borrow money from them. I guess your friends aren't telling you, Paula, so someone has to. Eh, Earl?"

Curt came into the bathroom when I was in there later. He asked, "Why do you want to wear so much makeup all over your face?" I said, "Oh, Curt, it's just what some people have to do. Hey, quick, what time is it? Want to ride bikes down to the beach and sit on our log and watch the sunset?" We did that a lot.

That was the year when I spent a bunch of Saturdays in a row at the University, getting dental work. The dentist would actually pick me up on his way downtown and take me to his students. My mom somehow found out they needed volunteers, so we didn't have to pay. I waited around and waited around in the reception area and they'd work me in between patients. My braces straightened everything out, but there still weren't enough teeth in there to fill all the gaps. "They're such little baby teeth," the dentist said. So they made porcelain teeth to cover up my tiny teeth and the pointy cones in the bottom.

Allen came by my locker at school. He was so big and hunky and had those tight T-shirt sleeves on his shoulders, so I never looked at him. I turned away, but he said, "Wait a minute, Paula, turn around, smile for me. Your teeth look gorgeous." He said, "Yeah, you have a beautiful smile."

Another day he said, "Seriously, Paula? You haven't been kissed before?"

"Nope."

He said, "That's the most astonishing thing." And, "I would like to show you how to kiss."

So I told him he could come over because my mom was going to work and my brother Greg would be gone with his friends and Curt goes to bed after his show's over. Later, we were in the kitchen. Allen turned me around by the waist and picked me up and sat me on the edge of the sink. He said, "You little feather-weight."

Our mouths were a little open. He showed me how to kiss. I was so happy to be doing that with someone. He was my first boyfriend. One afternoon, he came over to watch TV while Mom was at work. He was going to stay and meet her when she got home. It was a cold springy day, and I wanted to snuggle, so I said, "Let's make a fire." He got the wood from the basement. We started pulling newspapers from the stack on the hearth and he said, "Oh my God."

I looked over and said, "Oh my God."

In between the news pages were little piles of cash, ones and fives and tens. They blended right in. I couldn't believe we almost burned them.

When my mom came home, Allen and I were laughing about the money in the tinder, and she laughed, too, which was a relief, because she hadn't laughed in a long time. She was shaking her head and said, "Well, Paula, what am I supposed to do? That pest will find it anywhere. I can't use the dresser or my purse or the bank, or the kitchen drawer or the basement boxes or the trunk of the car. It can't be anywhere!"

She said she was going to take a bath, and not to snoop around too much more. As soon as she went down the hall we started looking under the couch cushions and behind the picture frames and even under my own mattress, laughing harder and harder because there was money hidden everywhere.

My dad showed up at my high school graduation. He hugged me in my gown and handed me a card and a little box. I took one look at him. Who knows how he got the money for something in a little jewel box like that? I thought maybe he traded his teeth for it. He hadn't been wearing them lately.

"Where did you get this, Dad?"

He said, "Well, that doesn't matter. Do you like it?"

It was a ring, with a pearl set in gold. It was very pretty, and I did like it.

He said to me, "I love you, Paula, and I'm very proud of you."

He looked so pathetic and skinny and sick. I wanted him to go before any of my friends saw us and came up and said, "Is this your grandpa? Can we see what he gave you?"

earl

I had to beg my ex-wife for cash. She thought I'd waste it, but I swore I wouldn't. I tried to explain to her in the simplest terms. "A man can't live like this," I told her. "I need groceries. I need medications. You force me to medicate on the streets, paying with anything I have."

On the farm when I was a child, despite his general shame, my father had given me a few useful things. Once when he was shaving, he delivered a piece of advice I didn't need until I was forty-one years old: "When a man loses his teeth," he said, "he grows whiskers to hide the shadows."

My brother Bud was making the trip to Betty's wedding all the way from Oregon. When he finally got me on the phone, he said, "Earl, you might as well come, too. It'll be all of us Hickman kids together again for Betty, bless her heart. Except of course Babe, rest her. Seven of us though, all on the farm again, God willing." He said, "I'm not sending you a check this time, mark me. But I'll tell you what: I'm buying an airplane ticket for you, and you can fly out and meet us in Cheyenne, and we'll drive from there to Sadie's. That dear. We'll all go out to the farm. Take it in again." I told him to send the ticket to Esta's address. He had no idea I lived at the YMCA, or what had happened.

When I landed in Cheyenne, my brother shook my hand strong. Even though I was a whole head taller than Bud and I had to duck to sit in the front seat, he couldn't look at me. Not when he shook my hand and not in the car. My brother never turned his head. But he somehow still seemed warm and smiling, happy to have me there. When we got to Sadie's, she came down the stoop clapping her hands. She stopped at me. Tears sprang up in her eyes, and she blinked fast and smiled and reached her arms around me. Then she stood back and shook her head, and finally she said, "Where's your teeth?"

She wanted to sweep me into her arms like a little baby. I could tell. She was like our mother living on, the maternal one of all my sisters. Seeing her just sent my mind to my mother holding me, and her rough hand on my head, rolling and rolling my hair the way I loved. I heard the camera shutter snap when we were all standing together next to Sadie's porch, just when I was pulling up my pants with my elbows out. "Like some old skinbird," my oldest brother laughed.

Before we ate, Sadie went to her youngest boy's closet and got out a belt and said to me in the hallway, "Earl, come over here and try this one."

She kissed me and patted my face with both of her hands. Reached up and touched my little skinny moustache with her pinky finger. That made both of us laugh.

I returned to Seattle and began a medical collaboration that made me feel as if someone really saw me. I was not a bad man. I was a smart, industrious man who kept falling ill. Fine doctors at the university hospital; they took an interest in my important case. They said I had something to offer. I went in for tests and evaluations over a period of time. And then, the day everything was in print, despite my pain, something in me came to peace.

The *Western Journal of Medicine,* spring 1974, had an entire article about me, although they never did reveal my name, as I requested, of course, given past situations. But there was my whole family pedigree drawn out, all the way from before my mother, with arms branching like marionette strings into my aunts and uncles, cousins, and me. Females were circles and males were squares. Strings hung down with affected males here and there: black squares, most of them with a slash through because they had died. In infancy. Of electrocution. By bullet unto himself. They died.

But I was there, in the center, at the bottom: the index case, the subject of the pedigree. The article was called "Case Report: Anhydrotic Ectodermal Dysplasia with Frequent Infections and Amyloidosis." Drs. Clark and Omenn, though mostly I had seen only Dr. Clark. It was drawn from clinic visits and patient files. How strange and wonderful it was to look back and see how they told it all:

> The index case is a 44-year-old unemployed chemist with anhydrotic ectodermal dysplasia, recurrent infections, and nephritic syndrome due to amyloidosis. Recurrent purulent and atrophic rhinitis has been present since childhood. Pneumonia occurred at ages 12 and 20 and recurred several times between ages 20 and 35. Recurrent cutaneous infections began at about age 30. The increased susceptibility to infections appeared to be related primarily to congenital factors. But some of the infections, particularly the episodes of cellulitis, were clearly related to subcutaneous self-administration of drugs. Amyloidosis, a previously unreported complication of anhydrotic ectodermal dysplasia, probably developed as a consequence of recurrent infections. Drug abuse has been a problem for 10 to 15 years and includes both oral and subcutaneous administration. Frequent psychiatric problems have arisen in relation to the drug usage. The patient is of normal

or higher intelligence and is well educated. Before the drug abuse began, he was a successful businessman.

It was simple, and it came from the pens of credible men. They published it to the world for me.

I could not remember what it was like to feel well, to be without pain. I felt a century old. My kidneys threatened to quit. They were turning me into a pillow of water waste, and so tired. But the article gave me new energy. I busied myself with the most important undertakings of my life. All day I made notes. Innovating, strategizing, keeping everything straight. Everything went on paper. Somewhere out of all those words, a plan would rise from the page—a way to the top. My research and development got very serious. The latest scientific technology. The grant funding available. I was ready. It was time. *Better root, hog. Or die.* There was very little I needed. Pens, lined paper, and library resources, including scientific documents and addresses for the highest government offices.

I didn't need to eat. I was absorbed in a feeding of a different kind: nourishment for my mind. Nothing felt better than the problem solving, the creating. There was so much innovation, and I wanted a part in it. For example, the day it said in the paper VEGETATION CAN BE A SOURCE OF UNLIMITED ENERGY. And a few days later, ANOTHER DAIRY PRODUCT: FERTILIZER. I thought of the dairy farms, and it came to me: What should we do with all that methane? I had heard President Carter when he said we had to stop relying on foreign energy sources and develop new, unconventional ones. And so, naturally, I extrapolated: Whoever found these new technologies would stand at the president's side, explaining, exalting, proclaiming that we would all be saved.

So, I abandoned my plans for an ambulatory lung clinic— respiratory therapy that comes to your doorstep in a specially equipped RV. I couldn't find enough grant money to get the vehicle. I also abandoned the work I had done to introduce an all-natural enzymatic substance for treating polluted harbors and docklands, as well as wastewater from manufacturing plants. I let all that go, and I focused everything on the future.

RE: Methanol: a very cheap fuel and clean-burning energy source.

Proposed: Use of human and animal waste for production of natural gas. Immediate environmental benefit: Elimination of pollution and production of high-grade fertilizer. Initial Research & Development* and Pilot project costing approximately $2 million, plus secondary $1.25 million grant will create a Net return of approx. $15–$18 million. Methanol produced by this process may be: a) converted to electrical energy, b) utilized as a fuel for transportation, c) employed for heating and cooling.

The final effluent from this process will be H_2O, which can be returned to fresh H_2O sources and reused. Other valuable by-products: highly nitrogenous fertilizer compound, and many other sophisticated biochemical compounds for consumer uses. (Unique as this last notation is, and I admit there is more conjecture expressed here than in the aforementioned material, my contention is that I would love to see this possibility for small-time entrepreneurial gains added to the total picture of R&D work to be done—and added with no ballyhoo. It's time Citizen Enterprise got a break.)

*Note: Much R&D work is already accomplished. Started in 1960 by Earl L. Hickman. I feel my work and accomplishments merit the money requested as a Grant-in-Aid. I would repay Social Security with some Grant funds. Or, for each investor dollar, a Gross return of $10 to $12 will be earned, with a Net return of at least 50–60 percent, which will assist and aid our ailing economy, plus provide badly needed energy, and eliminate some serious ecological problems. Even if the net return should fall to 25–30 percent, investments would still realize a sound return.

And so, when critics say it's impossible to endeavor to become completely self-reliant from foreign energy sources, I say: Scientific Technology and American Ingenuity will prevail! I read the headlines. "Consumer Energy Costs to Exceed Inflation Rate"? This need not be! John Q. Consumer does not deserve that treatment. So, how to avoid high energy costs? Ask me: Earl L. Hickman.

All of this, between my doctors' appointments and dialysis and trips to the pharmacy. I got into Social Security housing, a new place called Roxbury House, and things were so much easier. I could walk from there to the store, in case I needed something like a shirt or milk.

Paula came into my apartment like springtime. It was like she brought air with her, caught in her hair and her sleeves, and I could smell her light brown leg skin. She smelled like a field. Or a light, windblown rain. She said, "Look, Dad, I brought you a few more things for your place. Do you have any thumb tacks?" Then she blew out the door like a leaf, and I was staring at a poster of the sky. Waiting for her, or anybody, to come back.

paula

I started going to Highline Community College. I was
finally doing my own thing for once, so even though I wasn't a
hotshot in high school, I was getting straight A's now. I was in
clubs, and I went to my classes, and I loved the things I was learning, and I had great teachers. On the first day of speech class, I
sat close to the front. There was a guy sitting behind me acting
like he didn't care about anything. He had wild, curly black hair
and a big moustache all the way to the corners of his mouth. He
was wearing a white undershirt and jeans. Guys could get away
with anything even though we girls had to spend forever to look
cute. He kind of looked like a convict, with his plain shirt and his
sideburns and the way he sat in his desk leaning back with one
arm stretched across the table and a pencil hanging in his hand
like an old cigarette. As if he had a thousand better places to be,
and he was just gracing us with his presence. But what a grace it
was. I started watching for him everywhere. One day, I saw him
in the library. I sat down right across from him, and I had no idea
why all my fear disappeared. I said, "Tom, want to go for a bike
ride in Seward Park on Sunday?" He kind of winked and said,
"Well, yeah. In fact, I'm an avid cyclist." He showed up at the

park with a brand-new bike. He was more of a car guy, and he'd gotten that bike just for our ride. He knew I knew it, too, so that was basically adorable.

My dad was getting a little more situated. He had finally gotten Social Security to cover an apartment for him, a little tiny room in this huge new group home. He called to see if I could come help him get it set up.

"At least I have a decent place to stay until your mother comes to her senses," he said. "The ball's in her court. It's up to her to bring the family back together now. So maybe in the meantime you could come to my apartment, and we could hang a few things on the walls. You have that touch. When you come, I can make us dinner. Oh, and Paula? I got the Medicaid, too. I put you down as my emergency contact."

My mom and I went together to see his apartment for the first time. He invited us to come for dinner, and for some reason she accepted. His place was so small and drab and square, and it didn't have a window. It made me feel awful. But Mom didn't seem surprised by it. He hadn't made any food for us at all. It seemed like he was waiting for us to help him fix the spaghetti sauce, like he had no idea how to do it. But maybe by that point his hands were so swollen and weak that he couldn't open the jar. I never knew what to think anymore.

We sat down at his little tiny table, the three of us. My mom's voice kept piping. She was trying to keep it cheerful. Hearing her do that let me know how one sort of person tries to keep her heart from breaking. I was more the type to just let it all out and cry.

I was picking things out for his place, and my place, too. I had moved out of my mom's house and gotten a little apartment in South Seattle near the college. It had lots of windows, and I kept thinking about my dad's horrible place without windows.

Tom and I went on dates all the time. We'd go see movies or

take walks on the beach or just stay in and eat and drink and watch TV. Once when I got back to my apartment after class, I checked my bedroom to see if the workman had come by to hook up the phone line. On my bed I saw a note: *Looking forward to seeing you tonight. Love, Jacques Bonet.* That was the champagne Tom and I liked to drink. I couldn't believe he would come by and leave a note right where the phone company guy could see it. He just laughed when I tried to yell at him. He twinkled his eyes and changed the subject: "By the way, my folks said they'd be glad to come for dinner."

Before his mom and dad came over, I looked around to see the apartment through their steady, loving Catholic eyes. Their loyal boy Tom, the athlete and smart and funny kid, dates a girl from this apartment. So, what would they see? *Okay, it's pretty big, and it has a nice deck and two bedrooms and two bathrooms, and between her and the roommate it is kept clean, and of course it's located near her place of education. Paula has the tiniest single bed, even smaller than a regular twin bed. From her girlhood. There's no way she and Tom could fit together on that thing. Very good.*

And there was also my father's cedar chest. The one we have upstairs now. My dad loved anything made out of beautiful wood, especially that color—redwood, cedar. I kept my Bible on the chest and two candles. It would be clear to Tom's parents where I prayed. They would have been right about everything except the bed.

I was reading for my class, and it was nice and quiet. There was a soft gray rain outside and crows cawing. Then the doorbell rang, and I thought it might be Tom, or his parents arriving early. But when I opened it, there was my mom, with a plastic cap keeping her hair dry. I was worried she'd stay. I said, "Oh, Mom, you didn't have to drive all the way down here."

She said, "Well, I thought I'd better see where you were living and make sure it's not some rathole or something. But it looks good. I brought you something." Maybe she'd noticed I sneaked a few towels from her linen closet. She only stayed a minute, handing me a box from the department store: a whole set of forks and knives and spoons. I didn't know why she was doing that for me, but it was just in time for dinner with Tom's parents.

I picked out a poster for my dad at the store—a big sunset on a black background, so it would be almost like looking out a window. I went up to his place, and we pinned it up along the entire wall next to the door. I liked what it said. It seemed like a good message for him:

WHAT WE ARE IS GOD'S GIFT TO US. WHAT WE BECOME
IS OUR GIFT TO GOD.

I took Tom walking at Gatewood Elementary, where I had gone to school when we moved from Cheyenne. He had such warm hands. I said, "Maybe after this we can go walk some more, down at the beach." The sun was going down. He straightened his arm, to stop me by the hand he was holding.

"Hey, Paula? What would you say if I asked you to marry me?"

Even bliss like that would get wrecked before I could enjoy all of it. Mom called when I was still giddy. She was just fuming. "What possesses him to call me? I told him he can call you kids, but I don't even want to hear about it. He kept collapsing in seizures, and then he tried to kill himself again."

I was so mad. "What did he do? Take fifty more pills than usual? Eat a whole pharmacy?"

I could see my life opening into new possibilities. I didn't have to stay bogged down in my dad's misery. There were going to be good things for me. But I didn't know how to get him out of my way. My wedding was coming up, and I wrote him a letter. I poured my whole heart into it.

Dear Dad,

There has come this time for honesty. As far as your paternal relationship with me goes, that cannot be denied. I am your daughter. I'm twenty-one and a half years old. But as Paula's "father," you have failed. There were six years of happiness, and if I count Greeley, eight years. That leaves thirteen years of nothing but bad examples, bad experiences, and bad memories. Thank you, Dad, for those first eight years. For giving me a taste of family life that was normal and happy.

Forgive me for my bitterness about the thirteen years of family life you deprived me of. Perhaps your life wasn't important to you—nor the lives you created—for you rejected us for Drugs. Throughout it all, I have loved you, not for being a good father, maybe for being a friend, but I'm wondering if it wasn't perhaps out of obligation and pity. But like I said—as you've shown with this last suicidal antic—your life obviously isn't important to you. But my life is very important to me. And this latest episode has caused me my last tears of anguish, pity, despair, hope, etc. No, Dad, you're not worth the frustration you cause. I have to think of myself now. I've give-give-given to you—in hope, in love, in prayer. And it's been futile. For no matter how much we care, the fact is: You don't.

I cannot respect you as a person because it shames and angers me how you can abuse your body as you have. In partaking in this evil pleasure of yours, you have ruined God's creation of Earl Lee Hickman. Will you be proud to stand in front of God? Can you say, "I've strived to serve you well"? Can you say, "Everything I've done I've tried to do for your glory"? No, you will have to say, "I failed you, Lord. I ruined my body, poisoned my mind, and trapped myself in an ugliness I can't escape." He will chastise you, Dad, which I think you need. And someday he will help you overcome this horror you've locked yourself into. I wish it could happen another way, but you've proven to be too weak. We haven't been able to support you enough.

I can no longer tolerate you as you are. I shall not subject myself to any more letdowns. Dad, you must know I love you. If for nothing else than your kindness and sensitivity. But I choose my friends for quality. As my father, you blew it. As my friend I must pass you by. I am thinking of my life and my joys to come. My upcoming marriage, my future children, etc. Until you can contribute to my joys rather than my sorrows, I don't want you to represent my family. This is a hurting time for us—but I had warned you. You blew it this last time. I'm closing our relationship because I have a life to lead. I'm not saying I'm giving up hope for you. I will continue to love and pray for you, but all will be done silently.

Greg has consented to walking me down the aisle at my wedding to Tom. I prefer not to have you present. I imagine this really hurts you. But Dad, your years of rejection have come to a head. Now in turn I reject you in this small way.

Love,
Paula

I gave the letter to my mom and asked her to deliver it to him, since I was cutting off contact. I wanted her to read it first, because I felt like she needed to know what I was doing.

But Dad kept calling me. I finally called my mom and said, "I don't get it. Can he not read? Why does Dad keep talking like he's coming to my wedding? Did I not make that clear?"

Finally she said, "Paula, I could never give that letter to him. No matter how horrid he's been."

She gave it back to me in a manila envelope, folded in half, and labeled in her beautiful cursive, *Paula Relates, Dad and Me.* Always so perfunctory. I don't know why I didn't go on and send the letter to him myself, but I guess I thought there must have been some wisdom in what my mom was doing.

So finally I took one of his calls. He asked how I was doing, and he asked me to come over and tell him about my new job. I'd gotten a great position with Boeing, with top security clearance. I took all kinds of dictation and typed letters. I did finally go over to my dad's, to bring him some things and tell him about my job. I'll never forget the way his eyes lit up, like I hadn't seen in a long time. They had been so dull. I kept telling him everything about Boeing. He was listening for once. He seemed alive. When I told him how much the company officers trusted me with their million-dollar documents, his eyes just jumped and flickered. It made me melt, and smile, and feel like a girl again. I loved to make him proud. I wanted to close my eyes to feel the tiny head pat I imagined. But then he said, "Well, I can't believe this, Paula. It's all too good to be true. You actually have access to a *typewriter*. Do you think you could type some things up for me?"

He seemed wasted away. His apartment smelled horrible, and I always felt like I should find out if they could give him a better room, something with a window he could open for ventilation at least. The air was awful. Then I looked around his little room, and I saw all of his piles and stacks of paper and the pop bottles and cups and plates and his clothes. He always tried to keep his clothes neat, but they were threadbare, and they didn't fit him. There was just no crisp way to fold clothes like that. It made me exhausted to think about moving him and all of those loose things. His trappings. So I didn't even inquire—he just stayed in the same unit. He was spending more and more time in the hospital, anyway. If it wasn't pneumonia it was a staph infection, or seizures, or losing a kidney, or shakes and spasms, or bleeding ulcers, or colitis, or appendicitis, or liver disease, or his gall bladder, or cellulitis and unexplained sores, or he would just run out of drugs, wherever he got them, which would make him crash, and so he had to go in—and then he could get more. He was becoming famous in the emergency rooms: the guy who looked way older than his age, who showed up with a portable TV and a little suitcase full of drug paraphernalia, who would neverthe-less deny any drug addiction except for an episode many years ago, and who would later be found singing in his hospital bed, little stowaway pills in his sleeves and coat pockets and the folds of the bedsheets beneath him, pills wherever they rolled as he tried to sneak them down.

I remember that suitcase he carried. He was so poor. When his briefcase broke, he started with this caramel brown suitcase. I knew there were drugs in the suitcase. I knew there were grand designs and notes written on yellow legal pads. I knew there were letters from Senator Magnuson and Scoop Jackson that politely told him that no, they would not be interested in pursuing his proposals for new energy sources. Sometimes there would be the sports page, or letters from his sisters. There were soda crackers and jellies from restaurants.

Those were the days when there was always a wistful look in his eyes that meant, "Do you still love me? Do you still see me as healthy and whole? There is still much more to come, and I can get over this hurdle, and you'll find me valuable and strong again."

I couldn't change him. I couldn't change what was in the suitcase. When you ask me these questions, I wish you could see how quickly everything comes to the surface. I am now older than my father was when he died. When I look back, it breaks my heart even more now than it did then.

There was nothing he loved more than seeing us kids. I felt like it was up to me to keep him alive. The way he smiled when he saw me was my clue to get past his broken reality and build an illusion that would help him get through another day. So I would smile and hug and chat and generally convey an air of normalcy.

He started calling all the time about the work he was doing. "Paula, can you come over and pick up some papers? I need you to type this stuff up for me at work tomorrow. I have to send them out—multiple copies."

I had my own mail to send: wedding invitations. But only one thing in the world seemed important to him.

"Address them to President J. E. Carter—very formal. Then copies to all of his staff, starting with Hamilton Jordan. Then: Mr. James Schlesinger, and the secretary of agriculture and the secretary of the interior, and Senator Warren G. Magnuson. Secretary of Commerce Rogers Morton. Followed by Scoop Jackson (Henry M.), who chairs the Committee on Energy and Natural Resources. Frank Pagnotta is in Energy Policy and Planning under the Executive Office of the President. And J. J. Brogan in Transportation and Energy Conservation. We can't miss anybody."

I helped him through things the best I could, without really understanding what was going on. "Dad, let's go over this. Let's say *attachment*, not *enclosure*. And you have to tell me how you want the little diagrams to look. Do I just draw in the arrows? I made the copies you wanted of the Enz-All brochures. And in the letter I inserted 'in order to provide insight as to my credibility' before you start talking about all the stuff you did in Greeley."

Then one day he called, so excited. "Paula, are you busy?" I opened my mouth to say I was sewing ribbon onto my wedding dress, but he just kept talking. "Let me read this whole thing to you—you're not going to believe this. It just came in the mail today. This is the beginning of something very, very big. Now listen. And you and Tom should be thinking about how you might like to be a part of this."

Dear Mr. Hickman:

Your letter to Secretary Morton regarding an energy project was forwarded by the Department of the Interior to this office for response. The benefits you listed in your letter as results of your energy project are very attractive; however, since you did not include any description of sources, processes, or products, we are unable to give you any substantive comments or recommendations. Regarding your request for travel and per diem funds for travel to Washington, our governing regulations do not provide for expenditures of this kind. If you wish to pursue the matter, we suggest you give us enough detailed description of your ideas to permit a useful evaluation.

Your interest in our energy future is appreciated.

Sincerely,

Edwin A. Kuhn

"And Paula, he's the associate assistant administrator of Energy Conversion for Energy Resource Development. Can you believe this? You better not go too far from the TV in the next few months, because it's going to be your dad on the evening news. You are going to be one very, very proud daughter. I'll get everything worked up in more detail to send back to Washington, D.C. If I give you a draft, can you type it up for me?"

At my wedding, I tried not to fall for that feeling again, that feeling of him being so proud of me. But I couldn't figure out what his ulterior motive would be for the way his skinny elbow was shaking and his face was quivering as he tried not to cry. He squeezed my arm into his side as we walked down the aisle. I saw my Tom waiting up there for me, and I knew as soon as I reached him, all the garbage of my life would be in the past. I wanted it to be the last time I worried about my dad, because now I was going to be busy giving my love to my husband. *What a waste*, I thought, *that I gave so much of it away already to this guy next to me.* He was so tall and unsteady. I felt like I was holding him up. He said softly, so softly I could barely hear him, "Baby Doll, you look so beautiful." Then his body took its own weight, and I felt like I was floating.

At seven weeks, I felt grateful for fall. I could wear looser clothing to cover my bloated middle. I wondered if the neighbors noticed that I hadn't been coming out of the house much, except for my solitary daily walks. Indoors, alone, I could hide my suddenly blotchy skin. I could conceal my careening appetite and my hourly bathroom visits. Something about fall made me feel warm and safe, too—autumn had always had that effect on me. It was the cozy-down part of the year, when withered, scraggly petunias gave over their turf to chrysanthemums, lawn mowing slowed, and sunsets toppled earlier and earlier into the afternoons. Dan was the only person I wanted to see.

My first prenatal appointment loomed. It would open a week during which I would need to tell my secret to strangers over and over again. Dan and I had interviewed midwives during the first weeks of the pregnancy, trying to find someone who seemed warm and understanding, not too "medical" when it came to normal pregnancies and birth, and supportive of our unconventional journey through conception.

The first midwife had been brusque. She seemed unmoved by our story, as if Dan and I were following an everyday path.

Another midwife had hesitated when I told her that our pregnancy might not come to term. I heard a change in her voice, so I said, "I hope you'd tell us if you'd be uncomfortable working with someone who might make choices you don't support."

"Well," she said, "I am pro-life. But that doesn't mean you wouldn't get good care from me. I just can't feel any differently than I do about abortion. Once I worked with a mom who found out that her baby would be born extremely sick, but she didn't do anything about it. She just couldn't. She didn't feel it was right."

Even though this midwife ran the only freestanding birth center within reach of our home—a beautiful historic home appointed like a bed-and-breakfast, perfect for the birth we had begun to envision—I knew the relationship wouldn't work.

Finally, we met Anne, a hospital-based midwife, and felt grateful for her sensitivity to our tentative pregnancy.

"We'll schedule your first checkup for seven weeks," she said after we first met. "That way, it'll be too early to check for a heartbeat. You may not want to hear that yet."

At the checkup, which was a prerequisite for our genetic testing, I talked more with Anne about the upcoming CVS. I wanted to be sure that we were testing as early as we possibly could—I didn't want to lose any time due to incorrect dating of our pregnancy. Even though I had been charting carefully and felt certain I knew when I had become pregnant, the only way Anne could reassure me was to suggest that I have an ultrasound to corroborate my chart. I had hoped to avoid unnecessary sonograms, particularly because the CVS itself would be performed under prolonged ultrasound exposure. But it was too easy to become swept up in the tide of prenatal routines in the hospital system. I agreed to go downstairs for a sonogram after my checkup with Anne. In a dopey way, I thought it sounded like it would be interesting, even a bit fun. In a changing closet, I stripped to my underwear, pulled on a hospital gown, and stood waiting. It never occurred to me to call Dan. I didn't see the significance, just yet, of taking such a step, or of taking it alone.

A young man—he seemed to be barely out of college— walked me to a dark room with a table and a computer screen. "Just get up here and pull up the gown," he said. "We'll see if we can find your baby through the abdominal wall. If it's too early, then we'll have to do this vaginally." His affect struck me as immature, and I felt wary. But I kept with my pattern and gave him the benefit of the doubt. He had no trouble spotting the baby through the abdomen.

"Why are you doing early dating?" he asked. I knew this question was a breach of my privacy according to hospital policy, but again, I second-guessed my gut instinct, which was to clam up.

"We're planning genetic testing for about eleven weeks," I said, "and we need to make sure we have the dates right."

"Why are you doing genetic testing?" he asked. Now I knew this was more than prying. He was challenging me.

"So we can see if the baby is healthy," I said, then closed my lips. My face had begun to burn.

"Well," he said, turning the computer screen toward me, "here is your baby." He looked at me with his eyebrows raised for emphasis. "This is the child you're talking about."

Suddenly, a watery thrum filled the room. He turned it up even louder.

"That is your baby's heartbeat," he said, as if I couldn't recognize it myself. I didn't want to give him the gratification of seeing my tears, but I had nowhere to hide my face. He sat in silence, keeping his gaze fixed on me, as the heartbeat whooshed around us. He let it play on, well after he had recorded its rate. Finally, he faded the sound slowly down.

"And here are pictures of your baby," he said, handing me

two filmy black-and-white printouts. "You can get dressed now."
He shut the door and left me alone.

I stared at the fuzzy lima bean in the pictures, feeling awful
that Dan had not been a part of our first ultrasound. It had all
happened so quickly. I hadn't realized how sad it would be, how
much I needed his protection, or how important that moment
could have been for him as a father. I hadn't known I would hear
a heartbeat. Just as the ultrasound technician hoped, I would be
unable to forget that rhythmic, underwater rushing.

Half an hour later, Dan picked me up from the clinic.

"Dan, I made a mistake," I said as I climbed into the car. I
reached for him. "I owe you an apology."

"What happened?"

I poured everything out: the experience with the technician,
the heartbeat, and the pictures.

"You have pictures?"

I handed them to him and watched his curious expression
soften as he took them in: two images of a white, fuzzy-edged
blob inside the round, black frame of my uterus.

"You can't see much," he said, with a hint of relief.

"I think it looks like a lima bean," I said.

"A bean," he agreed.

"You should have been there," I said. "I'm sorry I did that
without you."

"It's okay," he said. "I would have liked to have been there. I
have to take care of my Kiddo. But it's okay."

In the following weeks, anytime I thought of the baby, a
rushing drumbeat filled my head. Although that sound had been
something I never intended to hear, and even though it had been
rudely forced on me, I wasn't sorry I had heard it. I couldn't help
but love it.

The following week at the dentist's office, I heard the drumbeat
again as I filled out the intake form. I hesitated on the patient

history. Should I mark that I was pregnant? I didn't want to talk about it. And I definitely didn't want to come back in six months for my next cleaning and have the staff wondering why my belly wasn't bulging. But I was due for x-rays and didn't want the exposure, so I scribbled it down: *Pregnant, 8 weeks.*

"Oh, that's the most wonderful thing!" the hygienist gushed as soon as she sat down next to me. "I'm just so, so happy for you." She was a rambler, and my mouth was occupied with instruments, so at least I didn't have to respond. Eventually, though, she wound her way to a monologue on birth defects. "When I was pregnant, they wanted me to take all those tests. You know, have an amniocentesis, all of that," she said. "My sister did, my friends did. Everybody does. And with my next pregnancy, I'm going to be in my later thirties, so I know everyone's going to want me to do it. I probably will. But I don't know what it's going to be like, all that waiting for results. My friend found out something was wrong with her baby but she had the baby anyway. That would be so hard. I mean, I don't know how I could ever deal with that. But don't get me wrong," she reassured me, looking down into my eyes through her protective goggles. "Even if something turned out to be wrong, I would never do anything about it. My husband doesn't believe in that. No one in my family does. I mean, I don't, either. We go to church."

She flossed my teeth, and I said nothing.

At home, I pulled out the lima bean pictures, precious yet burdensome. After showing them to Dan, I had tucked them into a drawer full of memorabilia. I wondered what I would do with them if the baby were not born. They were clearly dated, and marked with my name. Would I throw them away, in an attempt to erase every painful trace? Would I keep them in a scrapbook or memento box, unmentioned, for my children to discover and ask about someday? I suspected I would. I had always been one to keep artifacts of my life, aware that their meaning could change if I gave them time.

"Who are you?" I asked the pictures.

I found myself hoping that our firstborn would have black hair like Dan. Did I want a boy or a girl? When I imagined the bean as a black-haired boy, I felt he was strange and exciting, rarefied. When I imagined a black-haired girl, I felt safe: The bean floating inside was a reassuring presence. A girl—imagine.

On my lake walks, I continued to fantasize about a normal pregnancy. My hopes had flown out of control. "We're pregnant," I would whisper gleefully to the breeze, practicing our announcement. "We're having a little girl!" Or, "It's a healthy baby boy!" Whenever I was unfocused—watching leaves swirling or a grebe family paddling on the chilly water—I heard myself announce a daughter.

I had been looking for signs of luck. One foggy afternoon, I saw a bald eagle—a rare sight in the city—swooping low as it chased two fast-beating coots across the water. The sooty little birds escaped, and somehow the whole scene carried a sense of fortune. The sight of the eagle alone was a stroke of luck, and its vulnerable little prey had at least one more blessed day to live.

Another morning, I spotted the juvenile loon I had claimed as my good-luck charm. He had been solitary, fishing on and off for weeks, on the northern half of the lake. I loved watching him fish—he would dive for almost a minute, then surface with a mouthful of ragged blackness from the bottom. As I passed his hunting ground, I saw an older woman resting on a bench, praising her sitting dog. "Good girl," she said sincerely to the retriever. "What a good girl you are."

Good girl, I thought. *A girl. If only.*

But then, on other days, the lake seemed cold and luckless. In the weeks before the water turned to thin ice, fishermen clumped along the shore, eager to make their final catches before ice augers were required. I felt hot air from their heat lamps as I passed, and I always glanced into their buckets. Most of the fishing was catch and release, but the glimmering creatures with their hooked mouths still turned my stomach. Perhaps childishly, I felt sorry for them. They reminded me of a summer camping trip my family had taken with family friends when I was in elementary school. Our fathers had given us fishing lessons from the edge of Pearrygin Lake, in Washington. As we watched, they reeled in a beautiful carp. The hook was embedded so obstinately in the fish's throat that our dads couldn't throw it back, and instead laid it on the shore. Giving no thought to the hook, I instead watched the iridescence of the fish's scales, refracting rainbows as if the creature had been dipped in amber oil. I watched the fish's lips, thick and luscious, as they cartoon kissed the air. *Smack.* The other dad crushed the fish's head with a sharp rock. It fluttered and twisted, flopping away. *Smack. Smack.*

"It's what he had to do," my father explained to me when I cried. "Otherwise that fish would have suffered."

"But it did suffer," I insisted.

"It would have suffered more."

With just a week to wait before the CVS procedure, Dan and I dreamed big for the weekend: London? Florence? A polar bear safari in northern Canada? The day before we planned to fly, Dan scanned flights for availability. He came home and announced, "Bozeman, Montana. Time to pack."

I had been feeling queasy—nervous about the test, and still bothered by morning sickness. I was ten weeks pregnant. Bozeman, not too far and not too strange, sounded perfect.

"You pick out a B-and-B," he said. "We'll just check out the mountains, take a hike, see what it's like. The flights are wide open."

That Saturday morning, we awoke to greet a band of sun-pink, snowy mountains filling the bank of windows in our room. I had slumbered without waking once—our getaways, it seemed, helped me release my worries and find peace. Dan had relaxed, too. Staring at the mountains made him feel the way I did when I watched the ocean: worshipful, serene, grateful. We gobbled a big breakfast, nabbed freshly baked cookies, and headed to the market to assemble a picnic lunch. As Dan drove and I held my stomach, our long, low rental car scudded and slipped up mountain roads that were alternately sludgy with mud, deep with snow, and slick with ice. It was mid-October. Forgetting that we would be hiking at eight thousand feet, we hadn't anticipated a snowy trail. It was slow going in our low-tops. My body felt tight and my head felt tired, but I couldn't help smiling as Dan led the way. *If he had a tail,* I thought, *he would be wagging it.* He was at home, happy in his element, and refreshed in a way I hadn't seen since before our pregnancy began. It wasn't cold—sun blazed through the ponderosas—and we took a few miles of trail at a pregnant lady's pace, which was also the pace, I decided, of a bear with a bladder infection. I stopped to pee every half hour.

We detoured to explore a handful of frozen waterfalls, then spread our picnic on a pair of boulders above Arch Falls for lunch. I held the peace I found at waking, a trusting acceptance that the pregnancy and its unknowns existed only inside my body, and was naturally more my burden than anyone else's. The test would be Monday, the day after our return. About two weeks after that, we would have results—boy or girl, then HED marker or none.

I was eating a ton. Down went my sandwich, then an apple, then chocolate. With every bite, I thought of the baby and the nutrition I was sending down. I was working on a granola bar when the thought struck me: After an abortion, mealtimes would be sad. It would feel so desolate, I thought, to eat for only myself again.

Later, we clambered over Silken Skein Falls, whose chutes of water were frozen into icy baleen. At the end of the day, on our way out of the woods and toward a hot pizza dinner, we stopped at one last river pool. Dusk fell. Blue-gray shadows appeared grainy at the foot of the wide, low cascade. Someone had constructed dozens of rock cairns on the slope next to us, tower after improbable tower. Dan tramped to the edge of the icy water, exploring a fallen log. I stopped, transfixed by the frosty rings encircling smooth, round river rocks. I felt a whisper rising: words for the baby. But I held them in my head. I didn't want to say too much to this child until I knew whether we would meet. *If I knew you were our baby*, I thought, *I would tell you that you were in the mountains in the snow and ice. I would tell you that you were in Bozeman on a sunny day when the Bearcats beat Weber State in football, and there was smoke on the horizon, and a pink sunrise on the peaks.*

Staring at the ancient river rocks, I had the sense that their white ice halos belonged to our baby. Was I supposed to do something? Dan wandered over and saw the mist in my eyes.

"What's the matter?" he asked.

"I'm ready for pizza and root beer," I said, mustering a little smile. Inside, I feared I was playing with fate. I couldn't shake the feeling that I had the power to jinx our baby, even though its genes had long since been determined.

The night before the test, I dreamed I became lost in the hospital corridors, unable to find the office where the procedure would take place. By the time I found my way, the doctor told me I was too late. My appointment had gone to someone else, and I had missed my chance to have my pregnancy tested.

When I woke up, I realized how eager I was to avail myself of this test. Even though I knew the procedure would be uncomfortable, the landmark day had arrived. I was unexpectedly giddy. My dream reminded me how much I always worried over unknowns. I liked to be able to picture situations before I walked

into them. I had read all about chorionic villus sampling. Since
the doctor would navigate a flexible tube through my uterus in
order to extract cells from the placenta, it was more invasive
than amniocentesis. But studies suggested that the risk of miscarriage was about the same: less than one in four hundred, with
the emphasis that a doctor's experience changes the odds. Our
doctor, Preston Williams, had been one of the earliest practitio-
ners of CVS, and had been performing the procedure for decades.
But for everything I had learned, I still couldn't imagine exactly
what the procedure would be like. Nonetheless, I felt cheer: *I got
here. I came this far.*

I caught a noon bus to meet Dan at the park-and-ride. Together
we made our way to the perinatology office, without being late
or getting lost. I changed into a hospital gown, and Dan sat next
to me as I settled down next to the ultrasound machine.

"You doing okay?" he asked.

I nodded. "You too?"

He nodded, bright-eyed but quiet.

Shannon, the ultrasound technician, couldn't have been
a more refreshing change from the moralist I had seen a few
weeks earlier. As she placed the transponder on my abdomen,
she asked gently, "Have you seen the baby before?"

"Not recently," I said. "Not very well."

She measured the heartbeat for only a split second, with the
volume turned low.

"I'm having some trouble seeing how we'll get to the placenta
today," she said. "Let's see what Dr. Williams says."

After looking at the position of my uterus on the screen, the
doctor—smooth mannered and gray in a confidence-inspiring
way—consulted with a nurse in the hallway.

"Everything's fine in there," he said when he returned to the
room, "but we're concerned that we won't be able to get a good
sample. Because of the position of the uterus, the baby is in the
way of the placenta, which is what I need to reach. If our attempt

today doesn't work, the positioning of your uterus probably won't change until later, and then an amniocentesis would make more sense."

"When would that be?" I asked, feeling my heart rate rising.

"About four weeks from now. So, you'll have to think about how you'd feel about doing an amniocentesis if this doesn't work."

"What choice is there?" I asked. Dr. Williams nodded, knowing my question was rhetorical. A nod came from the nurse, too—a round-faced, warm woman who reminded us of Beverly, our genetic counselor from Iowa.

I looked at Dan. Neither of us had known that there was a chance the testing could be delayed. I had been so grateful I wouldn't need to wait for amniocentesis. I didn't want my pregnancy to begin showing, and I was mentally unprepared for an extra month of waiting. But instead of defeat, I felt a sudden surge of confidence. "I've got my fingers crossed that this is going to work," I said, practically ordering the doctor to give it his best shot.

"Let's get started," he said.

Into the stirrups went my feet, and down came the swabs of germ killer. I glanced at Dan, wondering what he thought. I supposed he had never seen a woman in the lithotomy position before—certainly not his wife. But his expression was calm. He seemed optimistic and kept leaning from his seat to see my face.

"How you doin', Kiddo?"

"Fine so far," I said.

The nurse unwrapped a long cannula, a thin, clear tube that would extend from a syringe in the doctor's hands all the way through my vagina and cervix, into the uterus with the baby and placenta. It might bump the gestational sac but would not perforate it or touch the baby.

"You're going to feel a pinch," the doctor said. "Bad words allowed."

He was placing a tool on my cervix, he said, to pry and hold it open. "Here we go."

I cringed, surprised by a shooting pain. It felt like a reckless pap smear. I breathed deeply, instinctively, through the sharpness. A moment later, I realized Dan was jabbing my arm.

"What are you doing?" I asked.

"Distracting you," he said. "See? It's working."

I smiled. The pain was almost gone, and I heard rapid sucking sounds as the doctor pumped the syringe, creating suction at the other end of the cannula in order to vacuum a sample of cells from the surface of my placenta.

Dan was transfixed by the screen, but I couldn't look. I focused on the space in front of my eyes, breathing carefully, afraid the pain might return. The doctor withdrew the tiny tube and checked the amount of tissue he had drawn into the syringe.

"That's not going to be enough," he said to the nurse. "Let's give it one more try."

I held my breath, but this time there was no pain. I turned to Dan, absurdly delighted.

"This time you have to watch the screen," Dan said softly, nodding encouragement. "Seriously."

I turned my head and saw the sonogram image of a thin plastic tube sliding into my womb, then snaking back between the baby and the placenta. And then, when Dr. Williams pumped the syringe, the cannula jerked like a garden hose gone berserk. Atop the hose, bouncing and spinning like a trapeze artist, was our baby.

"That kid is flipping all over the place," I said, somewhere between hilarity and terror. But the doctor didn't seem concerned. It looked like a dangerous ride, but judging by the doctor's lack of response, when you're that small and tucked in a sac within a sac within a womb, a few 360-degree whirls were no big deal. I found myself laughing. Dan joined in. It felt so good to giggle, watching our dumpling bob and spin.

Moments later, the doctor came to my side. "We got a terrific sample," he said. "More than enough, and it's perfectly clean—not a trace of maternal cells. You can go to the bathroom now, if you need to."

In the bathroom, I looked at myself in the mirror. My face seemed small and far away, as if I were a photograph of a photograph. I took a deep, ragged breath and began to cry. I was so relieved. Dropping my shoulders, I let the day's tension go. I took big dry breaths as tears streamed down, and I felt tightness leaving my body. The weeks of waiting. The months of wondering. The years of searching. "Almost there," I whispered to my faraway reflection. "You're almost there."

Back in the exam room, I asked the doctor if I could see the sample he had retrieved.

"I knew you'd ask that," Dan said, smiling. "Always the investigator."

"I always encourage people to take a look," the doctor said as he gestured for us to join him at the microscope. "Chorionic villi—they're really beautiful."

Even without magnification, I could see the tiny peach-colored fibers lying like sweater lint in a petri dish on the counter. A few more strands rested on a slide under the microscope. Our baby's genetic information lay tucked within those gangly filaments. Under the microscope, they were thick and fuzzy, like loose tufts of shag carpet. A few pieces branched like coral. They glowed tangerine. "They *are* beautiful," I said.

Dan held my hand through the parking garage. I felt overjoyed. I was relieved that I would not have to wait four more weeks for a test. I felt blessed that the sample had been clean and plentiful. And I knew wonder: Our bitty bouncing offspring had brought us together and made us laugh.

At home, I was thirsty for fresh air. The backyard beckoned. It was a warm October afternoon, flooded with golden light. A poky wind stirred, hinting that a chilly night lay ahead. Dan had an hour before he needed to head to the airport for a business trip.

"But I have time," he said.

"For what?" I asked.

"Don't you want to carve these pumpkins?"

I scrambled inside to gather up markers, knives, and scoops, then met Dan in the leaf-strewn grass. He propped our three pumpkins in a row, then stretched a trash bag for their innards between two patio chairs. I imagined what we looked like as we worked: two soft-skinned children in grown-up bodies and old sweaters with rolled-up sleeves. We crouched over our masterpieces, carving quickly in the fading light. An unaccountable gladness filled my chest. I couldn't contain it. I smiled without reason, feeling pleasure seep from my skin and wisp away in the clean air. I felt a balance: I had prepared for parenthood as much as I had prepared to let go. *I can wait,* I realized. *Now I know I can wait.*

I was wearing a red bathrobe, about to get dressed and catch the bus to go teach a writing class, when the phone rang two weeks later. Dan was at work. UNKNOWN CALLER, UNKNOWN NUMBER. I knew what that meant.

"We won't have the HED results for a while yet," the genetic counselor was quick to say. "But we have some preliminary information, and so far the other chromosome tests have come back normal. We also have the sex of the baby. Do you want to know that?"

I hesitated, unsure of any reason why not: A boy would simply mean we kept waiting, and a girl would mean all was well.

"Of course," I said.

"It's a girl," she said, her voice lifting. "A little girl."

I hung up the phone. Energy burst from every part of me. All I could do was pace quickly and crazily, my feet pounding the wood floor of the upstairs hallway. I breathed in a happy panic, alternating between chatter and sobs. I flopped on my bed, grabbed the cat by the ruff of his neck, and said, panting, "It's a girl. It's a girl. It's a girl. You're going to have a sister."

Finally I stopped, pulled open my robe, and looked down at the small swelling of my belly. "Hello," I said. "You're a girl."

As I dressed, all the little hopes I had held in check began surfacing. I could choose the words to tell Dan, that night at dinner. And yes, we would have a baby to match the age of the neighbor babies due around the same time. I could tell my parents they would have a grandchild. I could tell Amanda and Luke that they would have a niece. I could call my friends. I could browse maternity clothes. I could let go. I could stop worrying. I could look ahead to childbirth. To motherhood.

I hurried to do my makeup so I wouldn't miss the bus. *What kind of idiot*, I asked myself, *does her makeup while she's crying?* But I smeared tears into my concealer anyway. I took a deep breath, composed myself, looked in the mirror, and said, "Now we can give her a name." Which naturally sent me over the edge again. Wet-faced, I dashed out the door. *It's a girl. It's a girl.*

The bus passed the Basilica of St. Mary as we rode into downtown. It was noon, and the bells clanged loud, round, and full. It was heraldry, celebration. I unleashed a fresh round of tears. Briefly, I paused to wonder how the tolling would have sounded if I had received bad news that day. But in truth, I thought, I probably would not have noticed the bells at all.

As I tried to teach that afternoon, I kept fantasizing about the moment when I would tell Dan the news. We happened to have a date planned: Japanese food, followed by a play. I envisioned us sitting down at the hibachi table. Pretending it was no big deal, I would say, as I shrugged off my jacket and draped it over the back of my chair, "Hey, the genetic counselor called today."

"Oh?" he would ask, suddenly stock-still, turning his eyes to meet mine. "What did she say?"

"It's a girl," I would answer, in a tone of triumph. "We did it."

We would embrace, and music would fill our joyful silence.

But by the time dinner rolled around, I had a splitting head-ache. I didn't quite strike the tones I had rehearsed. "It's a girl," I did finally blurt, just as the chef invited us to order.

We chose our flavors and watched him cook. Our silence was nothing like the one I had imagined.

"A girl?" Dan asked.

"We're having a baby," I said.

Dan nodded and swallowed, watching the chef toss our meat to the side and throw our vegetables into the searing heat.

"This is good news," I said, unsure what was happening.

He turned to look at me. "I knew everything would be okay," he said. "But I always thought it would be a boy. It never crossed my mind—"

My eyes filled with tears, but I asked more questions, trying to understand. Our dinner conversation was calm: stories from Dan about how, as an only child, his only model of fatherhood had been male to male. He told me how much he loved playing with his dad as he grew up, and said he felt stumped by the sud-den need to reimagine fatherhood.

"I'm sorry, it's just going to take me a while to picture everything."

"I'm tired of waiting," I said.

"I know," he answered, returning an untouched bite of sushi to his plate. "Just a little longer."

I thought I could be patient. But later, during the play, as my headache grew worse, my reasonableness melted into anger. On the car ride home, we barely spoke.

The next evening after work, Dan waltzed through the front door in a chatty mood. *Can't he see I'm still upset?* I wondered. He tried tickling me, teasing me, asking about my day. Finally I said, "I'm not in the same mood you are."

His movements came to rest, and he said, "All right, Kiddo.

Listen. It's not that I'm not excited. It just wasn't the news I was expecting."

He walked back to the porch and brought something inside.

"Surprises are supposed to wait until after dinner," he said, "but here."

Dan had never been the type to apologize with flowers or speak through gifts, so when he handed me a bagful of presents, I was done for. Cinnamon rolls, movie tickets, and zoo passes—all things he wanted to enjoy with me. Then I grinned as I unwrapped a bright pink maternity shirt that announced COMING THIS SPRING.

"I'm taking you back to Seattle this weekend," he said. "We'll surprise our parents, do all our announcements in person."

I wore my new pink shirt on the plane. Just after we landed, I dialed Luke. We wanted to tell him first. He took my call, even though it was Saturday night and he was surrounded by friends, migrating with the crowd after a college basketball game.

"We won," he shouted into the phone. "We're celebrating tonight!"

"I called to give you something else to celebrate," I said.

He let out a whoop, knowing. But he let me tell him anyway. "You're going to be an uncle," I said. "You'll have a niece this spring."

His shouts reached Dan in the driver's seat. "I'm gonna be an uncle!" he hollered, grabbing his friends, calling their names, telling one after another.

"After everything you've gone though," he finally said into the phone. But I could only think of his own struggles in that moment, much more real than my own.

"You're going to be the best uncle in the world," I said, trying not to cry.

"I *know*," he yelled. "I'm gonna be awesome!"

* * *

The genetic counselor had promised to call again two weeks later, when she received the HED results and could say whether our baby girl was a carrier like me. Only after that call—long after—did it occur to me that I could have chosen not to receive that information. A girl; that was all we really needed to know. But at the time, even though our daughter was nearly certain to be symptom-free, it seemed natural to allow the testing to continue. Before we received the results, Dan and I decided that no matter what the news, we wouldn't share it beyond our family. Just as I had chosen to tell him, years before, the risks involved if we were to have children, the choice of whether to discuss their genes belonged to our children: the one we would soon have, and the ones we still hoped for.

part four

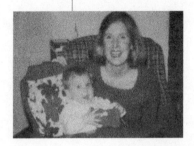

Bonnie and Paula in Redmond, Washington,
1979

Josephine came with perfect health. She was a carbon copy of her father: dark-haired and bump-nosed and long-toed and sweet-lipped and loud. She was also an imprint of me: wide-awake exhausted, strong-willed, intent, and eager.

Dan had quickly become the father I had always imagined for my children: focused, attached, eternally good-humored. He showed me how to be respectful of our daughter's every flicker of identity. Hurrying back from work each evening to scoop Josephine into his arms, I could see he felt at home only when the three of us were together. Josephine had been with us a few weeks when Dan told me he could hardly wait for her sibling—or siblings.

When Josephine was nine months old, the sand hills of Nebraska thawed on the first day of March under record high temperatures. From its low angle, the sun mustered mighty waves of white light. We climbed out of the car in the Kimball Cemetery, stretching in the warmth, leaving our coats—two big, one tiny—deep in the trunk. Just in time for our visit, the heat had melted the snowdrifts that had covered the Hickman family graves all winter. Only a few white patches remained on the grass.

We had taken the highways from the Denver airport, exclaiming at the long, straight roads. Windmills, antelope, missile silos, a broad horizon over endless yellow grassland; everything refreshed our perspective—we had been hunkered down in our cold corner of Minneapolis for too many months. Passing within a few miles of Greeley, I felt an unnerving proximity to the past, yet I welcomed the discomfort. I was still in the process of recording the past, and it had become history to me too— almost flattened like the pages of a book. But the locus of those stories stirred me again. Now, instead of simply remembering Earl, Esta, my mother as a girl, and even Junior, I felt them again. It was an old, familiar chill in my blood. A sensation entirely known, yet transient, like a swallow in the throat.

At the cemetery, where my grandfather Earl and his parents rested, I felt the tug. I unbuckled baby Josephine and carried her toward the graves. Dan followed with the camera, trying to give us space, trying to let this be, for a moment, about only us: a single shoot from a distinct branch of a particular family tree.

The cemetery snowplows had sprayed Earl's grave with gravel and clods of turf. I brushed the pebbles and dirt from his rough stone, glad to rub it, swipe after swipe, with my wide-open palm. Becoming a mother had shown me that sometimes practical gestures were even more loving than sentimental ones.

I felt wary. I didn't want to use my child as a prop. I didn't want to place her in an artificial context and belabor her every sweet gesture with too much meaning. It hadn't bothered me to prop her against the gravestone of her namesake, her great-great-grandmother Josephine, but I felt differently at the side of Earl's headstone. I remembered my mother's story about taking me, a one-year-old, to visit Earl. He was sick again and she wanted to cheer him up, so she hoisted my little body onto his bed. He winced, burdened. I didn't want to do this to him again, but at the same time, I felt what my mother must have felt that day almost thirty years earlier: *Look! Look what I did!*

I kept Josephine to the side of Earl's headstone, holding her close to my knees.

"Do you know who this is?" I asked her. "This is your great-grandfather. He was a special man. He's part of our story. He's part of the reason you're here."

No more words came to me. Dan, watching from a few feet away, said, "Let her say hello."

She had learned to wave. Together, we waved at Earl, and at Josephine, and at the other Hickmans around us. With Dan's encouragement, I loosened my grip on our daughter, letting her stand, holding my fingers.

"Stand back," Dan said as he crouched with the camera.

I steadied her, then pulled away my hands. She reached, balanced, stood.

Sadie had been waiting for us, eager to meet the little girl named after her mother. Josephine sat on her lap, playing with her blouse buttons. Sadie, camera shy, hid her face when we tried to take a picture. But after dinner, she emerged from her bedroom, dressed in red and dabbed with lipstick.

"What a lovely scent," I added to my compliments.

"It's just hand lotion," she said shyly. Then she handed me a disposable camera and asked me to take her picture with the baby.

"You're my little doll baby," she said to the girl on her lap. "My little doll baby, Josephine."

I snapped the photos.

"My mother would be so proud," Sadie said.

"Of what?" I asked.

"Of this," she said. "My mother loved the little babies."

The next morning, we awoke to a blizzard. Josephine watched from the living room sofa as Dan shoveled Sadie's driveway.

As soon as he moved the snow, a new layer took its place. We crawled back to the airport along the highway, catching glimpses of the road between billows of white. I had never seen tumble-weed blowing with snowdrifts. Josephine slept. In that car, we were so warm.

paula

Tom and I were expecting you. We were renting this little
yellow cabin down on the South Sound, and we got your crib all
ready. We loved having people come over for parties on our lawn.
It was summer. On the Fourth of July, your due date, everybody was drinking beer and barbecuing and looking out over the
water. I told Tom, "You better come with me—I'm going to have
this baby." He looked surprised and said, "What?"

I said, "Come on, we're taking the boat out. This kid's going
to be born on the Fourth of July if I have anything to do with it.
I want to see if I can bounce it out."

He just sat there in the boat terrified, holding on, but laughing, too. I stood in a straddle and slammed across every wake I
could find out there. But you hung on five more days, including
one and a half of labor. At the hospital, they pulled you out with
forceps and left a bump on the left side of your head. I tried
to kill the doctor for hurting you, never mind me. I guess I've
always been that way.

After we got home, Mom drove Curt and Dad all the way
down to the cabin to visit us and see you. I will never forget how
my dad looked at you the first time he saw you. He held you on

his lap and rolled his spine in a curve over you. In that moment
he had the softest eyes I ever saw, big and brown. Even though
he was emaciated, his face and hands were puffy from edema.
His kidneys were failing. Maybe it was his big round cheeks and
tiny smile that gave him that soft look. His swollen hands held
you steady, and he just smiled that gentle smile for a full minute.
Then he whispered, "I've been waiting to meet you."

When he said that, I felt like something gently clicked in
me—something left swinging wide open a long time before.
That day, he gave you the pink blanket you carried around all
those years. I made chicken for dinner, and I was the last one to
sit down. When I cut my meat, I saw it wasn't even cooked. "Oh,
shoot, everybody give me your meat. It's not done."

But my dad had already finished most of his, and his mouth
was full and he was chewing joyfully. He said, "No, no no no, it's
fine! You did a great job on it." I took away his last bite so I could
finish cooking it. When I sat back down, I checked on you while
your dad held you at the table. My husband, my Tom. I was so
proud to be married to such a good man. And I was really proud
of you. You were still just brand-new, and you had these long,
skinny legs. I said, "You're so lucky, Bonnie. What a good papa
you have. What a good papa."

Then my dad's head jerked up and his eyes got bright and he
looked right at my mom and said, "Paw paw?"

She started to smile.

In a singsong he said, "Where oh where is the dear little baby?
The dear little baby?"

I looked at you, and I looked at Tom. My mom was shaking
her head like, "Oh, now don't start this, you clown."

Then Dad took a deep breath and started singing: "A-wellll,
away down yonder in the paw paw patch, the paw paw patch!"

My mom started to laugh through her nose. He leaned over
toward her and said into her ear, "Picka paw paw, put it in your
pocket."

She finally burst out laughing and said, "Oh, Earl, *stop* it!"

The two of them kept hoo-hawing like lunatics. Tom and I just looked at each other. At least they were happy. They stayed like that the whole night.

I loved nursing you. When my milk went into you, I could feel this love just getting more and more powerful. As though it filled us both from the very core out to our skin. I said to my mom at one point, "You know, I really get this bonding thing now. You didn't breastfeed me, did you?"

"Oh, *whshh*," she said. "We just didn't do that. Nobody was doing that back then."

Whenever you slept, I smashed bugs. There were big black ants and termites in that place. I couldn't stand the thought of one of those things crawling on your perfect skin. I went around the floors and the walls with napkins, *thump, thump, thump,* trying not to wake you up.

My dad would call. "Paula, are you busy? Oh, a poopy diaper? Well, just listen to this real quick. I just got the most amazing and wonderful letter from Warren G. Magnuson. Do you want to hear it? You won't believe the tone he takes, Paula. The way he sees me as his partner in this struggle. It's just so promising. Okay, so listen." And he'd read another letter that was courteous but nothing more.

With you every day, my mind filled with colors. Toys and swings and finger paints. I planted seeds for all the funniest flowers I could think of, sunflowers and cosmos and poppies and floppy-headed bright drowsy things. I could just picture the way you were going to laugh at the way all those colors bobbed in the wind when they opened, and you were going to take your first steps among the blooms. We would read and sing and dance. We would go riding in the VW with the top down. The whole life I wanted arrived in my eyes.

Seven months after we visited Earl's gravesite with Josephine, I began hearing that whooshing sound, like a sea cave in my head. Everything had scent—layers of scent. There were dreams. On a Saturday morning in October, my father was visiting as he passed through town for a business trip. He sat at the dining room table, sharing his oatmeal with Josephine. Upstairs, I took a moment alone with Dan.

"This is weird," I told him. "I think I might be pregnant again."

"Really?" He got in the shower. While he scrubbed behind the curtain, I peed on a stick. I was unsure what I wanted to see. One line meant not pregnant, two lines meant pregnant. I watched grains of pink begin to blotch the little window.

"Dan?" I asked, watching the stick, willing myself uncertain, "is that two lines?"

Toweling off, he glanced over. "Oh, absolutely," he said, utterly nonchalant.

"That means I'm pregnant."

"I know," he said.

I was quiet. Relying too much on intuition and not enough on data, I had misjudged my cycle. Our intention had been to wait at least until Josephine was two before we considered another baby. I had just restocked our rack with beautiful wines and set a pound of good strong coffee in the pantry. All of my maternity clothes were out on loan. I had just gotten back into my slimmest pre-pregnancy jeans. I had been quietly looking forward to a time when my body would be my own again. Josephine was sixteen months old and in the process of weaning. We had just finished one home remodel and were about to begin another. It seemed we might be moving the following spring, due to changes in the airline industry. Maybe Atlanta. Maybe Europe. We loved the adventure of Dan's job, but it was a peripatetic lifestyle. I was unsure how a second baby, so soon, would fit in. If Dan shared all of these uncertainties—not unlike the uncertainties that he had borne alone the first time—how could I endure another tentative pregnancy? I needed him to be on board this time, so he could bring me with him.

A few feet away in the bedroom, Dan practically hummed as he dressed. I could see his reflection from where I stood. He wore more than a hint of a smile.

Josephine called us from downstairs. I turned to Dan as he passed down the hall, ready for the day.

"Is this okay?" I asked him.

Now fully beaming, he said, "This'll be fun."

"It's fine?"

"It's fine, Kiddo." He smiled and bounded down the stairs.

I stood staring into the bathroom sink, not ready to see my own reflection. I was grateful for Dan's spirit, but ready to let the subject drop. This time, I wasn't so sure I wanted to talk about it. I preferred to take our daughter to look at the ducks or play on the swings. I knew I would tell my sister, but I already knew I wouldn't need to talk with her about it every day. Instead, I wanted to tell her about the piecrust recipe I had found and Josephine's newest words. Anything but dwelling on the unknown.

That morning, we went to a little farmer's market in the

neighborhood. While my father carried Josephine around, exclaiming at pumpkins and searching for mango juice, Dan came to my side.

"You're pregnant," he said, nudging me.

"You're excited," I answered, charmed by the pleasure dancing in the corners of his mouth.

"I know the timing seems a little crazy, with the possibility of moving right before the baby would be born," he said. "But I was thinking it also might be great. Maybe perfect."

"I know what you mean," I said.

"Do you think it's a boy or a girl?"

"It's probably a boy," I said. "We couldn't have timed it any better if we tried."

His smile made me smile.

"Okay then," he said, taking a deep breath. "It's fifty-fifty."

The once-quiet, misery-making mornings of pregnancy, in which my lonely mind spun out of control with worry and confusion, were now crazy making in new and wonderful ways: baby class and autumn walks, toddler colds and diaper fights, sliding at the park on sunny days and playdates at the coffeehouse when it rained. I told none of my girlfriends about my pregnancy, but I leaned on them nonetheless—they kept me afloat by helping me to have ordinary days. Whatever I would reveal to them after three months passed, I knew my friends would understand the way I had relied on them to distract myself from my secret. Many were pregnant themselves, and I distantly missed sharing every tiny detail of the experience. But I knew better.

I scheduled our CVS for mid-November, making sure to avoid any extra appointments, tests, or consults. At my eight-week checkup, the midwife asked me whether I wanted to hear the baby's heartbeat.

"Sure," I said, falling into my old pattern.

She left to find a Doppler scanner, the handheld sonogram

machine that would play the sound of the heartbeat into the room.

What am I thinking? I asked myself in my moment alone on the exam table. I felt my feet and hands go cold, my armpits moisten, and my heart begin to race. I felt choked and nervous— I wanted to change my mind, but something made me afraid to announce this. *Rehearse,* I told myself.

So, only to myself in the quiet room, I said, "I changed my mind about hearing the heartbeat." The words flattened the lump in my throat so I could say them again, easily, when the smiling midwife returned.

"No problem," she said, moving on.

When I left the appointment, I felt the same, emotionally, as I had when I first walked in: peaceful, calm, happy, sane. I had maintained my integrity, and this felt like an accomplishment. From there I knew I would allow no ultrasounds before the CVS, and there would be no lima bean pictures to haunt my drawer. I felt so different this time—motherhood had made my protective instincts decisive. I knew if I didn't take care of myself, I would not be able to take care of anyone else. Feeling cheerful, I drove home through a wet snow, excited to make a pumpkin pie with Josephine.

Physically, I felt on top of the world. Even though I needed extra naps, I felt strong, fit, and energetic as I shopped, cooked, rotated laundry, planted bulbs, wrote, and played with my daughter. I had gained too much with my first pregnancy, so I watched my weight carefully this time. It was just another way in which I felt more in control of my life and body; pregnancy was not simply happening to me. I chose to be with it, awkward though it sometimes was. Each Wednesday night at dinnertime, I walked out the front door and up the hill to the elementary school library, where, between bookshelves and filmstrip reels, I unrolled my yoga mat for an hour of community-education heaven. I knew the other neighborhood women in my state were taking prenatal yoga classes at a different studio. But in the school library, surrounded by both men and women, spotting the spine of *Pippi Longstocking* for balance, I felt strong, safe, and protected exactly where I was.

My peace of mind was not entirely manufactured by force of will. There was something deep down that told me I could be calm. I was sure our baby was a boy, which was exciting even though it could just as well have been scary. I was also sure he was healthy.

Over pasta in an Italian restaurant in the neighborhood, on one of our rare date nights, Dan and I both confided our relief that the pregnancy had been unplanned.

"It just got handed to us," I said.

"It's better that way," he said.

"We weren't responsible for choosing the right egg, the right month, the right day."

"And if it works out, it's just a blessing," he said.

Finishing each other's sentences, we were not only on the same page, but also on the same line.

As we walked to the movies after dinner, Dan experimented out loud: "'A family of four.' Hard to imagine. It'd be fun."

"I really feel like everything is fine in there, Dan."

"Good," he said, taking my hand as we walked.

Distraction continued to work. I busied myself with planning a Halloween party for the neighborhood kids, organizing a writing workshop, and attending my first three births as a doula. Over the course of my first pregnancy and Josephine's arrival, I had feasted on studies and stories about nature's intentions for childbirth, learning countless benefits of good births for mothers, babies, and families. I signed up for birth-doula training, and Amanda found the same calling. More often than we chatted about my new pregnancy, we rehashed the latest news in maternity care and traded tips for supporting birthing women. At the same time that I enjoyed the diversion, it was also a reminder of my condition. A surprise breech had made the home birth I planned for Josephine into a cesarean. I felt eager for another chance at a natural childbirth.

I resisted games of superstition as much as possible. But one cold morning, I turned the ignition to no avail. "Come on, come on, work this time," I said out loud as I turned the key again. I heard my words as a command to the new pregnancy. There was a blessed rumble to life.

Some nights, after our long, busy days, it did take me a long time to fall asleep. The unknowns found me there, lying on my back, watching the night shadows on the ceiling. I let myself work on the hard questions then: *What is my worst fear? What if I have an abortion? How will I feel?* I would lay one nervous hand on my still-flat abdomen and the other on my heart, as I had learned to do in prenatal yoga with Josephine. With deep breaths, my optimism would return, and then I could sleep.

My dreams brought strange and beautiful and sad things. One night I awoke after a wise woman had delivered an enormous truth about my pregnancy. But as soon as I opened my eyes in the dark bedroom, her words were gone. I lay there, listening to my daughter's deep breaths in the next room. Knowing how ardently I monitored her breathing as I slept, I felt a sudden sadness for my own mother. I missed her, and I now understood that all my life, as I moved farther and farther away, geographically and personally, she missed me—her sleeping-baby me—more than I had ever known.

Warm October sun gave way to a thin November chill, and fresh-air walks with Dan and Josephine kept me feeling light and energized. One afternoon, as Josephine slept in her stroller, Dan and I talked about the upcoming CVS.

"When is it again?" he asked.

"End of next week," I said.

"Already."

"I know. It's been so peaceful this time."

"So much easier," he said.

"I think I could do this again," I said. "We wouldn't have to stop at two kids, you know. I love having a family with you. We're still young. Maybe we'll have more."

We trudged up Queen Avenue, pushing the stroller, breathing the thin, cold air.

"More and more, it seems so perfect," Dan said.

"What instructions should we give after the test?" I asked. "Should they call us while we're in Italy?"

We had decided to take another trip alone together after the testing was done. We planned a week in Italy, and Josephine would stay in Minneapolis with her grandparents. It was the first time we would leave her. As much as we dreaded separating from her, we knew we should give ourselves—and our daughter—a release from the tension that would surely fill the house as we waited for the phone to ring.

We stopped for hot tea and continued our walk home with the cups warming our hands. We decided our genetic counselor should call us with any news up to the day of our departure—we thought we would find out the baby's sex before then—and then not contact us at all during our week away, no matter what. If she received news that I was carrying a boy affected with HED, we asked that she schedule my procedure, and call me on our return with the date and time. I found myself beginning to wish for relief from the strain of waiting. What if it was a girl? Our trip abroad would be a celebration—not just an escape. But I was getting ahead of myself.

It was becoming clear that there was a good possibility we would be moving soon. We didn't talk about it much, because each day the news from Dan's office was different. One day, we faced the idea of moving to the South in about a year. Another day, it would be a move overseas, within the next three months. With all of the uncertainty, it was possible to let the move slide into the background; it was a likelihood, but without places or dates it didn't seem real. But one night I dreamed that Dan said to me, very clearly, "I don't know if you really understand this, but we are going to need to leave here in just a few months."

It was another wait-and-see to carry.

Two days before the CVS, in the midst of a real-life roof replacement, I dreamed of house and home. In the dream, I walked across the street to take a look at the roofers' progress, and I was shocked to see that they had torn off the front of the house upstairs. I could see straight into my office, with my messy desk and unmade-scrapbook piles and rumpled futon couch. The roofers explained that irregularities in the roofline—undulations we had actually discussed in real life—were caused by twisted timbers in the walls. They had to strip everything back and start from deep inside in order to make everything right on top. I felt out of sorts, because I hadn't asked them to do this work. I just wanted them to roof right over the bumps because a deep solution was far too much work. Still, I had a sense of calm, knowing everything would be better in the end, and so I told them to go forward. In spite of the fact that the neighbors had a view of my whole personal inner mess—and I could not access that area while the work was being done—I was surprisingly at peace.

But I awoke unsettled. I knew that a dream about a house is a dream about the self. I was tired of living a lie around my friends, intentionally keeping from them the very sort of thing we always shared. Perhaps the dream was reflecting a yearning for the inside to match the outside. Or did I want the outside to reflect what was inside? I had been so certain that all was well with this pregnancy. Perhaps I needed to simply trust myself and skip the test altogether. I didn't like the way the impending test seemed to disturb my growing baby's peace, but I was far from certain that my intuition was right about which genes the baby had inherited. We would go forward with the test, but I realized I needed to reassure the baby. *It's going to be bumpy,* I silently said. *But Mommy and Daddy think this is important to do.* I needed to persist in believing, so that my body would keep telling the baby that all was well.

"Everything has been so painless this time," Dan said as we drove to the CVS appointment a few days later. "We already know where to go, what to expect. Now we just have to get this last part over with." I felt giddy once again. *We made it,* I kept thinking. Maybe the test days were so jubilant for me because they were a date I could count on, close to the end of the tentative period. But also, I knew, I might never have allowed myself to become pregnant if the testing had not been an option.

The CVS itself, with the same doctor and the same nurses, fit the pattern of the pregnancy as a whole: far less painful than the first time, with a wait so quick that it was over almost before I realized it had begun. While the doctor took a sample of chorionic villi with a quick draw of the syringe, I stared at the ultrasound screen.

"There he is," I said. The picture was a perfect side profile. I immediately loved the little face I saw. "He's moving his arms and legs."

Dan watched the screen in silence, not tempering my certitude that we had a boy.

And then there was the heartbeat, more powerful than the visual image, more profound and lovely and terrifying in its perfect pace.

"All done," Dr. Williams said.

"Anticlimactic," Dan said, smiling.

Dan and I had a moment of privacy in the room as the doctor took the sample down the hall. "He looked great to me," I said quietly, referring to the image we had seen. Already, I was looking forward to a birth. In the testing room, I made no effort to mitigate my hopes. Maybe I felt I had less to lose; we had a child already—a flawless, funny, brilliant one. Anything more would be an embarrassment of riches.

We would have complete results by the beginning of December, with the possibility of having the baby's sex confirmed before we left for Italy in the last week of November. But a week after the CVS, having received no news of any kind, we kissed Josephine goodbye, boarded our plane, and turned off our phones.

We jam-packed our trip, spending nights in four different areas of Tuscany. We walked tiny towns and vineyards. We puttered in our rental car through orange-leaf woods, wondering if the farmers who had parked their old cars along the roadside were hunting boar or truffles, or both. In Vernazza we admired citrus and olive trees, sharing cappuccinos beside a crashing sea. We drove through snowy Apuane Alps, returning to warm autumn as we dropped back into the valleys. Near Lucca we got lost trying to find which hill to hike in order to find our high-perched inn. We overate for dinner, overate for breakfast, then walked among fig and pomegranate trees. In San Gimignano, we climbed to the tip of the village, out early and alone on a sparkling morning. I asked Dan to take my picture as I sat on a castle wall. In the picture, I sat sidesaddle on the wall, holding a gold scarf tightly in my hands, awash in morning sun, with a smile both sheepish and glad. Later, a drive to Florence, the whole of which was sheer nausea for me. In the city we returned our rental car and ate sublimely smooth gelato served from a chocolate shop. We watched a rainbow settle over limestone facades. We marched from sight to sight, talked with Josephine on the phone, and took delicious late-afternoon naps. On Thanksgiving Day, we climbed 463 steps to the top of the Florence Cathedral's Duomo, working up an appetite for yet another feast. I loved being back in Europe, and I was happy to be so busily exploring and partaking of the ancient, traditional, and delectable, all so easy to find. But in truth, I couldn't wait to go home. One reason we traveled was for adventure, but I was craving routine. My heart and head were already overfull of the unknown and unexpected. I was ready for the test results. Even as we drove through Tuscan villages and autumn's brittle bosks, even as we entered magnificent cathedrals and strolled along crumbling country walls, even as we hiked cliffs high above the sea and stared at David's huge hands, I struggled to find inspiration.

On a rainy afternoon, we found ourselves trudging the city. With drenched jeans and a sodden umbrella, we climbed a few steps to the long, covered loggia at the front of the Ospedale degli Innocenti, a six-hundred-year-old foundling hospital. Reliefs of swaddled babies hung between the archways above us. At the end of the long corridor was a railed-off niche in the wall. Until the late eighteen hundreds, it had held a wheel—I imagined like a small playground merry-go-round—where unwanted babies could be left. The wheel was designed to rotate the baby into the warm interior of the orphanage without revealing its parent's identity. On the wall above the wheel was a Latin inscription, taken from Psalms: "Our father and mother have forsaken us; the Lord has taken us in." My eyes smarted; I had come a long way, but still, guilt was never far off. Neither was the sense of the word *innocents* in politics. But just then, as we stood tired and far from home in a gray November rain, my heart ached not only for the innocents but also for the fathers and mothers who bent beneath those words of shame, placed their offspring on the *ruota*, and touched them for the last time.

paula

Around the time you learned to walk, I got you all dressed up and I made sure your hair was curled and you were fed and clean and happy. I put you in the car with me and we drove over to see my dad in the nursing home where he was staying for a while. I had lipstick on, and I was dressed up, too. I kept picturing the smile that was going to come over his face when he saw you, his doll of a granddaughter. Just like the first time he saw you. I would have given anything to be in the presence of that smile again. I just knew you were going to warm his heart; he was going to be so tickled. I liked to make people happy.

All the nurses saw us going by, and they said the nicest things—"Oh, ohh, you two! You both look so beautiful!" We went into his room. Before I said anything, I held you up so he could see your little face and your hair and your whole outfit, even your little shoes. He looked over at us, and all he did was blink. I stared back. There was hardly any spark in his eyes. I said, "Dad, look, we're here. Look who's here."

He said, "Hi," rasping. So I took you and I tried to kind of straddle you over the top of him, so he could see you right there above him, all the charm and sweet innocence in the world, descending like an angel. But he winced when I put you down on him, like he couldn't handle the weight of you. Our presence itself seemed like too much.

I wondered what was wrong with him. I simply wanted to show him this little girl I made. When you and I left and walked down the hall, I know those nurses were making sad faces behind us. They could see how wonderful we were, but my own father couldn't. When we got home, I called Tom at work. He said, "Peej, are you crying again?" He listened to me tell the whole thing about how it went with my dad, and finally he said, "Paula, you know I'm at work and I want to, but I can't always help you with this stuff. Not every single time."

I started writing some poems when you were sleeping. And when you were awake, we sang. I loved to sing to you. *You are my sunshine, my only sunshine, you make me happy, when skies are gray . . .*

You were learning to talk, and you would say along with me, "S-sine. S-sine."

I sang to you all the time. *I'll always love you and make you happy, if you will always stay the same . . .* I sang while I was getting you dressed one morning, and when I finally stood you up, you took your hand and put it over my mouth and said, "Don't sing, Mama." I know I shouldn't have let it hurt my feelings.

At the weekend market, I looked over a display of beautiful canes. Carved of twisting red wood, they seemed almost braided. I looked at the different shades and finishes. They had interesting things for handles, like a length of bone or a knob of elk horn. I stood there feeling them with my fingertips. It was fall and starting to get chilly. It dawned on me distantly: Wood never got too hot in the sun, and it didn't get too cold either, even out in a frost. No wonder my dad loved wood. I ordered the perfect cane for him.

"My dad is tall," I told the carver finally. "He can't stand upright anymore. How soon can you finish it?"

earl

Dear Mr. Kuhn:

Elaboration: The scientific principle in "overall proposal" is as old as time itself. The designed, much-desired end result is the [check Roget's Thesaurus] combination/combobulation (whatever) of: a) Solid proven scientific formula, and b) Feasible and economically sound phase-out of reliance on fossil-derived petrochemicals. See Formula, below.

SCIENTIFIC FORMULA

Sun: the #1 energy source →

Earth →

Plant + Original Life →

Food production: x # of Calories = x # of Energy →

Man: Emerging work produced by Mankind: Waste contains x # of Calories →

When waste is treated, x # of Calories = x # Energy in the form of methane or methanol →

Methanol from waste (or x Calories) = x units methanol, convertible to x amount energy.

I liken this revolutionary formula to the discovery of a new element or chemical compound. I call this compound The New Molecule. It is so new that its molecular configuration and the bonds, linkage, is just beginning to evolve. Call me the Do-Or-Die Molecule! I use the chemical molecule only as an analogy, an illustration, because it graphically demonstrates how bonds hold things together—every tiny part is important. A stable chemical compound requires each molecule to be in its place. You can really see the importance of this metaphor as a parallel to the intricacies of a functional energy program.

Goals: Search
And Research.
The answer is very plain: A Cycle. God's Way.
Father Time + Mother Nature are not together. She started with diet pills (now called Speed, Uppers). She's hooked, thanks to modern medicine and so-called advanced technology. And now, alcohol. Depressants. We—you and I—are mostly responsible for Mother Nature's sad state. For decades, we have aided and abetted her addiction. Things are in a hell of a mess. But until Mom and Dad (Father and Mother) are reunited, our environment will stay a mess. And to Historians, that is our story: Our scientists and technologists and doctors—how stupid can they be? We scientists, we doctors who care, are responsible for Mother Nature's condition. We know the environmental problems are actually compounded—worsened—by the separation and divorce idea. We are trying to treat Mother Nature so she can get back with Father Time. It is a very difficult thing to accomplish. We were so bright! A man shot. Actually, we were very immature—yes, even childish. Showing off. The answer is very plain.

Sincerely,
Earl L. Hickman

Nobel Prize: Certainty of winning.
Projected Salary: Minimum $180,000. Possibly millions.

It is the best work I have ever done. Your mom is so puffed up with pride in her father. And I've been feeling better—now the kind doctors, they all believe my pain. They mix them like drinks for me: pain cocktails, we all call them. I can have them at home. And I feel like the king of a sailing club, where the wind is always blowing, and the sails go *snap snap snap*, and the gulls swarm all around the boats, but never mine. Mine so fast and winning.

paula

My dad kept asking me to type up his notes, but he was getting weirder and weirder. Sometimes I had to just tell him I would type everything up and mail it for him. He was so happy and expectant, like he knew his dreams were all about to come true. But physically he was falling apart. He was out of it more and more of the time, and he kept having strange accidents. I got a call that he was in the hospital again—this time he had walked right through a floor-to-ceiling windowpane when he was leaving a store. He just somehow missed the door. When I saw him in the emergency room, he had a hundred little cuts and scratches—not just the usual sores on his legs. He had lost a ton of blood. I couldn't help thinking about all the work they put into keeping his blood clean with dialysis, just spilled on the sidewalk in front of Fred Meyer.

Later I picked him up for a dialysis appointment. He was standing there in the sun, wearing a pajama shirt, and trousers that wouldn't stay up, and his tiny little jacket didn't even fit him over the pajamas. Where did he even get a jacket that small? He got into the car and said, "Hey, Baby Doll," like nothing was the matter. I looked at him. His face was swollen, but overall he was a ghost of bones.

The news came on the anniversary of my grandfather's death. It was a Tuesday evening, two days after our return from Italy, the eighteenth day of our post-CVS wait, and the thirteenth week of my pregnancy. That morning, I had destroyed my cell phone by sending it through the laundry in my coat pocket. It was as if I had made a subconscious shift, dreading the sound of a ring. Our genetic counselor had told us a few days after our return from Italy that, indeed, I was pregnant with a boy. "Okay, that's actually what we were expecting, so no surprise there," I had said, not realizing how crazy I must have sounded in my cheerful acceptance of the fact. But, not missing a beat, she promised to call as soon as she had results of the HED screening.

It had been thirty-six hours since that conversation. As another 5:00 PM close-of-business passed, I resigned myself to at least one more restless night's sleep and set to work preparing dinner. Josephine played in the basement with her grandparents, who were scheduled to depart the next day.

The phone rang. My hands were busy—chopping vegetables, perhaps, or stirring a pot—and I missed the call. I didn't stop to check who had dialed us. I didn't bother to look for a message. I let myself pretend this was not happening. But by the time the phone rang again half an hour later, just as Dan pulled into the driveway, I knew I had to face it.

"Bonnie, I'm afraid I have some bad news," our genetic counselor said. "The baby is affected."

My ears exploded with a clanging sound that drowned out her voice and the soft rushing of my pregnancy. Dan walked through the front door to see me skidding toward him in my socks, holding the phone to my ear, stricken. "What is it, Kiddo?" he asked.

"Bad news," I croaked, pointing at my belly, hearing nothing from the receiver pressed to my ear.

He pulled me in. My eyes closed against his shirt, and he held my head between his chest and arm. Slowly, with deep breaths, I began to hear bits of the words coming through. Procedure Saturday. Doctor will call. So, so sorry.

Lifting my head to look at Dan, I saw the same wet, red eyes I remembered from the day we found out that I was a carrier. The sadness in his expression was as much compassion as disappointment. With the phone still in my hand, I felt the ground beneath my feet and took my weight from Dan's arms. Just then, I was flooded with a feeling I never could have expected: gratitude. An enormous wave of thankfulness for the fact that I could know, then and there, that the faulty gene I carried had passed to the one in my womb. Science, technology, and the gentle care of strangers had opened for me a possibility my ancestors could never have imagined.

Now, a far more difficult test was about to begin. A trial of our planning, of my conjecture about what I would want, and of my prognostication about how I would feel. Before I even hung up the phone, I felt a deep sorrow for the little life I carried. But I did not waver. Our plans still felt like the best choice we had.

The genetic counselor had left a message with the earlier call I missed, so the details I needed were preserved for me. I could

listen again later, when I was ready to write everything down.
Logistically speaking, the hardest part was the delay I now faced.
Minnesota law required me to confirm my consent for the procedure at least twenty-four hours in advance—which meant that
legally, the soonest the procedure could be scheduled was Thursday
morning. But the doctor would be at a conference Thursday and
Friday. She couldn't help us any sooner than Saturday morning,
when she would be kind enough to get up early on a weekend
and come to surgery. That night, we told Dan's parents I needed a
hospital procedure later in the week, and they quickly agreed to
extend their stay to help care for Josephine—and really, all three
of us.

When I spoke with the doctor the next morning as I gave my
consent and discussed the procedure, she apologized for the timing
problem and condemned the state law. "It could be over by now,"
she said.

"Don't tell me that," I snapped. "It's too hard."

In the three days I had left, I had more decisions to make.
Preparing me for what to expect, the doctor mentioned that I
could choose between heavy sedation and general anesthesia.
With heavy sedation, I could breathe for myself and wake up
immediately after, but I would have no memory of what happened. General anesthesia would put my mind and body to sleep
and have a longer-lasting effect. Most women, she said, chose
sedation over anesthesia.

"Isn't there another option?" I asked. "I'm just thinking, I've
done a lot of work to really face what is happening here, and I
feel like I need to honor myself and this baby by making this
choice in full awareness. I'm afraid if I sleep through it, I won't
really be owning up to what's happening."

She paused. "We could just do a spinal," she said. "You'd just
be numb from the waist down and completely conscious."

"I need to think about that," I said. "I think a spinal really might be best. I'm afraid if I miss what happens, I'll be haunted by the gap."

"I understand," she said. "But keep in mind, you might have the same problem if you witness it."

"I know," I said.

"For now, I'll write down that you want spinal anesthesia and nothing else, and you can always change your mind."

"One more question," I said. "If I took the sedatives, would the baby get them, too?"

"We don't know," she said. "We just don't know the answer to that."

I called off two meetings. I canceled a phone interview. I left calls and e-mails from friends unanswered. I was spent. For the next few days, I did something I had been afraid of: I disappeared from my daily life, and I knew all the neighbors and friends who were used to seeing me out and about could tell something had happened. I wondered how, and when, I would explain myself. In a moment of wisdom before a marathon nap, I made a choice: Outside of our parents and my sister, I would not tell anyone about my pregnancy, or the loss of it, until at least four more weeks had passed. This would give me time to feel out exactly which people I really wanted to tell, and how I would talk about it. The period of raw pain, I hoped, would be brief enough to keep private. If I still felt emotionally ragged after the holidays had passed, then I would know I needed more support. Somehow I knew that I would feel safest grieving in privacy, at least in the near term.

The work of that grief began that night after dinner. Dan withdrew into a game of tickle-and-chase with Josephine, and I went upstairs. In bed, I pulled the covers over my head, smashed my face into a pillow, and allowed a different kind of cry: ugly and uncontrolled. When I was too tired for more, something told me that after three such awful purges, I would be better again.

* * *

Thursday morning, when it was still dark, I opened my eyes into a lucid dream. It was a different way of understanding that death comes, not an idea, but a shiver, a prickling of hair, an iron-and-mineral taste of blood and bone. In one horrible instant, I perceived the distinct reality of the loss to come: a tiny fetus, forced through the small opening of my cervix, losing its form. The termination of my pregnancy was not just a concept, to be discussed and decided. It was flesh and reality, life and loss—an empirical subtraction. It would create a tiny change in the hard and physical universe: a shift in mass, more real than the weight-lessness of thought and sentiment.

Lying there in the early dark, with two more days to wait, I felt my body continuing to grow our tiny son. *It is just so hard,* I heard myself say. But still, it did not feel wrong. I did not wish to change my mind.

I shuffled to the kitchen, heavy-lidded. Josephine and her grandma were getting started with the day's breakfast. My mother-in-law took one look at me and suggested I go back to bed. I did just that, grateful for the chance to pass a few more timeless hours. My morning nap brought another dream. This time, I was with Dan and Josephine in a beautiful Italian village near where we had stayed on the first night of our trip. I was expected somewhere, for a ceremony of some kind. But things were taking longer than usual, keeping us from embarking. We had to cross to another village by a narrow cliffside trail over-hanging the sea. Each time I stepped onto the trail, vertigo was so strong that I feared I would fall over the edge and die. I kept returning to the beginning of the path, where I felt safe. Trying again, the swirl of dizziness was so powerful that it felt as if my body was being pushed over the edge. Finally, I crouched to look over the edge. It was a long way down—but I realized it wasn't as far as I thought. I realized that even if I fell, I could survive the splash and swim to shore.

I might not have gotten out of bed again that day, but I heard my daughter giggling as she played with her grandmother at the bottom of the stairs. I pushed off the covers and thumped slowly downstairs. There was my girl, her hair sweetly rumpled, dressed in an adorable clash of stripes and flowers. After Saturday, this was what would be left for me: my plentiful home, my healthy family, my happy child. *I just have to get through it, and then everything will be fine,* I told myself. Everything I had read warned me to prepare myself for the emotional aftermath of an abortion. The hardest part, it was said, came after. I would be heartbroken and confused. I would experience the loss in unexpected ways. Was it wishful, I wondered, to hope that my years of learning, planning, preparation, painstaking choices, and cultivated self-respect could deliver me from that aftermath? I imagined returning to my house on a cold December morning to sit with my child by the glowing Christmas tree, saddened but unbroken.

That afternoon, the phone rang again—yet another in the parade of calls I both welcomed and dreaded as I took care of consent, planning, medical history, hospital intake, and other details. This time, it was a kindly nurse who worked with the doctor. Most of the conversation was review, along with some standard security questions. She asked me to confirm my name and birth date, address and phone number. And then she asked, "In your own words, what is going to be done on Saturday?"

Like a schoolgirl about to recite a poem, I took a deep breath and dutifully began: "I am going to—" And then I froze.

The nurse waited as I tried to find my breath. In my paralysis, generations of family flashed through my mind. Stories I knew and stories I still didn't quite understand. The knowns and unknowns of HED. My brother's dazzling mind and tender eyes. A baby smile I would never see. The graveside explanation I had attempted for my grandfather. The rationale I still couldn't articulate clearly enough to give my own mother. What would be done on Saturday? Abortion, termination, interruption, D&E or D&C, ending a pregnancy; no word had quite the right sense, and no word could hold enough. I could not deliver any one of those simple terms without the chance to tell my whole story.

Finally I asked, "Do I have to answer that?"

"It's just for security," the nurse said softly, "but no, we can skip that."

"I guess you know I know," I said.

By Friday morning, with just one more day to wait, I saw the light at the end of the tunnel. Even though I still felt bone tired, I actually wanted to get out of bed. I went out grocery shopping, stocking the cupboards with a week's worth of healthy food. In the afternoon, I donned my red-striped holiday apron and set to work baking molasses crinkles and Russian teacakes, my December favorites.

I had always hoped for a prompt procedure if a pregnancy tested positive for HED, nervous I might suddenly be repulsed by the idea of continuing to grow and nurture a baby that I did not expect to meet. I imagined that I might even be repelled by his tiny presence. But instead, I continued to feel of a piece with the physical pregnancy, in a still place between embrace and relinquishment.

The act of baking for my family had been a comfort, even though I'd had no appetite to eat any of the cookies. But then, after dinner, I had a sudden panic: These cookies were something I gave in love and warmth to my family every year, and the boy inside me was family. So I ate a few. And then, panic bubbled up again. We had only a few hours left. What else should I do for the baby in his life with me?

"Something you like. Something that makes you happy," my sister said when I called her with that awful question.

The best I could do was to walk down the stairs to the basement, where Dan was romping with Josephine on the carpet. I simply watched them play. The few times I laughed, the sounds were true. Before bed, I was to bathe in antiseptic and give myself clean sheets. As I slid down between them, knowing my long wait was all but over, I turned to dig in my nightstand for a pen and a sticky note. *Dear Son of Ours,* I wrote. *Is there any way you could ever understand that I am drowning in love for you?*

paula

When I got the news, it felt like a thousand doves flying out of me, free. Greg and I were supposed to pick his casket. We had to pay for it ourselves, and money was tight, so we had to be reasonable. We knew Dad liked pretty wood, so we looked at the rich deep reds and browns, cherry and mahogany; we knew not to get pine, because that was just your basic cheap funeral. We didn't really know what questions to ask or what to do when you picked out a coffin, so I just ran my fingers along the sides, and every once in a while, I guess I thumped one like a cantaloupe. We saw one that was shiny and nice. It sounded heavy and solid. I looked at Greg. He shrugged and said he thought it was fine, too. We wanted to make sure it was long enough, since Dad was so tall. When we asked about that, the funeral home guy in his little gray suit waved his hands like, "Don't worry, don't worry, we always check that." Then he took us around into the office and said, "Now, an obituary for the paper is included in the price of arrangements. Would you like to write it now?"

The man went away and we were sitting there with paper and pens and a sample write-up. After all the vital statistics—*Earl Lee Hickman, 49 years old, born in Bushnell, Nebraska*—and all of his relatives' names, there was one paragraph where we could add something unique about him. Greg and I just sat there. There was too much to say, and too little. Finally I asked, "Well, what did he do?" We thought about all the diagrams and drawings in the letters he'd asked me to type up. We remembered the illustrations in his patent applications, and all the papers he moved from Cheyenne to Seattle in place of Mom's china. All the big plans he always had. In the end, we decided to just say: *He was an art designer for medical products.*

When I took down the poster I hung in his apartment, I wondered about the gift God now had before him: Little Earl Lee, wasted away. I shuffled out all of my dad's papers and papers and papers, and then I came to his clothes. I had to pick out a suit for him to wear, so before I got rid of anything, I pushed through the odd pieces hanging in his closet. Back against the wall, I found some sea-blue trousers I always liked, soft and bright. They went with one of the jackets. There was a patterned shirt that matched pretty well. And a tie—I thought maybe a bright one for a little splash of color. He always did that when he could. When I held up the pants and the jacket, I realized they were probably too big. Maybe they were his clothes from back in Colorado, where I was still in love with him. Maybe that was why I liked that outfit so much. I thought since they were in the closet, maybe there was a chance they did still fit. And anyway, I figured if something was a little big, they could just pin it underneath him. My dad's side of the family always did open caskets, but Greg and I decided to keep it closed for the service in Seattle, before we put him on the plane to Nebraska for the funeral out there.

Pastor Brown asked us kids a hundred questions before the service. We knew he'd do a decent job for Dad. He asked us if we wanted to say anything, and I thought, *Like what?* Every story ended with a disappointment. Greg and I just looked at each other, thinking along the same lines: *He basically killed himself with all those drugs.* His autopsy said he experienced fatal arrhythmia due to kidney failure, and the kidney problems were due to amyloidosis. The amyloidosis was secondary to infection. But which infections? The ones his condition never spared him, like pneumonia? Or the ones he arguably caused himself, from chemical burns, needle jabs, and accidents? It was as hard as ever for us to tell where our dad's condition ended and his intentions began.

We left you with Tom's mom, so in the church it was just me and Tom, Greg and Curt, Tom's dad, and a couple of other relatives. My mom had gotten dressed up and met us in the funeral home before the service. But when it was time to go into the church, she just stopped.

"Mom, aren't you coming?" I asked. She stood frozen for a minute. Then she turned around and walked back to her car. I never asked her why she didn't go to the funeral. I guess it didn't surprise me; she just wasn't a part of things then. Greg and I were left to make Dad's arrangements ourselves.

In the church, I looked around at the measly little crowd and thought, *Okay, so here's the moment of truth, and the verdict is in: My father was such a loser that apparently he's not even worth remembering.* I started to feel embarrassed by my dad all over again. He kept that power to shame me.

I heard Pastor Brown say, "and Earl was a man of great talent, of many accomplishments," and I leaned over so Greg and Curt could hear me whisper, "Yeah, like stacking potato chips."

Tom's dad shot me a look, so then I felt bad, but still not the right kind of bad.

At the airport, they told me where to walk out to accompany the casket, and where to watch the plane take off. I stood in the wet wind while they put him into the cargo hold. I waited there until he started flying, the wheels picking up and folding, his little cross of gray slipping up through the mist. It was cold, but

I kept standing there. I was thinking about when he called me, right before he died in his apartment. He said, "Hey, you'll never believe what happened."

"What?"

"They asked me to be in the choir!"

I said, "You can sing?"

He said, "What do you mean?"

"I just didn't know you could sing."

"Of course I can," he said. And then his voice dropped down to the proudest, happiest little whisper. "And Paula, guess what?"

"What?"

"They want me to sing a solo."

◐

Snow fell in the dark as Dan and I drove to the hospital. Our car made the first tracks in an inch of white. Pink cones of light flared from the streetlamps, filled with tumbling flakes—the kind that glittered like sequins in the headlights before tires sent them scattering. I was struck by how beautiful it was in the dark and cold. I felt alone in the city with only Dan, and the two of us leaned on each other, subdued and heavy, strong and certain.

"Dan?"

"Yeah, Kiddo?" He said softly, looking over at me. His wool hat covered his ears and eyebrows, and his ski coat was zipped to just beneath his nose. His eyes caught the street's swirling glow.

I asked, "Is this the hardest thing we've ever done?"

He thought for a moment and said, "I don't know."

"I don't either," I said.

More silence passed. "Is it the saddest thing we've ever done?" I asked.

"Yes," he said.

We parked in the ramp and walked toward the main entrance of the hospital, two down-bundled figures arm in arm in the dark. The hospital was quiet. The surgery floor was vacant except for one nurse who came down the corridors to find us, already knowing my name. Paperwork began, question after question.

"Do you have any questions for me?" the nurse finally asked.

"I'm wondering how often this surgery happens here. For genetic reasons."

"All the time," she said. "Every day. Yesterday, there were three." She paused. "I've been through it myself."

After intake came the part of the morning I dreaded the most: the moment when, by placing in my cheek a drug that would open my cervix, I would begin my own miscarriage. Dan sat next to me, red-eyed. We met with the doctor, an obstetrician who was a matter-of-fact, yet perhaps a bit battle-weary, supporter of reproductive rights. The anesthesiologist would arrive next. I had talked it over with Dan and decided finally that I wanted to be sedated—to sleep through the procedure and to allow the sedative's amnesic effect to take from my mind any possibility of a memory. I had been reflecting on the choices I had made to protect myself from too much exposure, too much information, in this second pregnancy. As much as I wanted to be accountable for the serious choices I had made, I also held the responsibility for protecting myself. I could own my choice without punishing myself for it.

The anesthesiologist placed an IV in the back of my hand, about to begin a wave of light sedation. As he worked, despite a room full of strangers, I lost my last self-consciousness and focused on my belly. I began rubbing and rubbing my abdomen with my free hand—a motion that would not end until I was deep asleep. My breaths turned to sobs.

"Bye, Dan," I managed, as they wheeled me toward surgery. And then, my focus went back to the baby at my center. *I love you. I love you. I love you,* I silently told him as I cried, trying to suffuse my womb with warmth. I paused to wonder whether there was anything more I needed to say to him, but there was not. *I love you. I love you. I love you.*

earl

Your mother lays you in my arms and I look into your face. *I've been waiting to meet you.* You open your eyes. You open your mouth. I think you might cry. But you don't make a sound.

After surgery, I woke up crying the same way I had gone under. It was as if the sedation had split my last sob in half. I finished it with a gasp, then looked around. Dan sat on one side of me, a nurse on the other. The sun was up, pouring rays into the room.

"I feel better," I said, announcing my first thought.

Dan nodded, smiling through a tired expression. It seemed I had just said a strange thing, so I checked in with myself. But it was true—I did feel better. Better than I had in days. Maybe even weeks.

"What did you do in the waiting room?" I asked Dan.

"Well," he said, clearing his throat, "I cried."

I was learning to stop asking too many questions, to stop trying to pinpoint Dan's emotions all the time—the precise thing he was sad about at what precise time, in what proportions. I understood that everything could simply be mixed up and overwhelming. I appreciated his tears, no matter which aspects of our ordeal felt saddest to him, and no matter how those compared to my own saddest parts. I felt so lucky to be loved by him.

I was unsteady on my feet, bleeding, and tender. Dan helped

me as I changed into my clothes, finding electrode patches on my skin and carefully unsticking them.

"Here's another one," he said, lifting my arm.

As we located those markers—the only evidence, besides my bleeding, that something had happened to my body in the hands of strangers—I stood amazed by the trust such a thing required. After all of my preparation, the last thing I had to do was to surrender and believe that I would be cared for.

Dan and I had agreed that we wanted a ritual to mark the day's passage. On the way home from the hospital, we stopped at our neighborhood gift shop and chose a painted, wooden Christmas ornament: a tiny blond boy, barely an inch tall, riding a flying goose. We would hang it together each year. It would help us remember, reflect, and be thankful for wherever we were and whoever we had become, individually and together as a family. When we walked through the front door carrying our little shopping bag, we heard Josephine playing downstairs with her grandma. We had the living room to ourselves, so we took our moment in front of the tree. We kissed, held hands, and I chose a branch.

Each day, I felt better than I had the day before. It was as I had hoped: With the procedure behind me, I healed swiftly and, it seemed, cleanly. I was content and excited to move on. The same wisdom that had protected me from self-torture throughout the pregnancy—keeping me from telling too many people, collecting ultrasound pictures, or lying awake through an abortion—soon revealed a safe, honest way to explain my recent disappearance to anyone who asked: I had lost a pregnancy. At thirteen weeks and two days.

It was strange and jarring to leave pregnancy without a birth. One moment, I would be driving from the grocery store to a coffee shop to do a little work, eating half a sandwich, thinking about nothing but deli turkey and traffic. The next moment, I would feel bereft: *Wasn't I missing something?* Remembering the specificity of the little spark that was gone, I would wonder, flicking on the windshield wipers, crumpling my sandwich wrapper, grabbing a drink of water, if his abandoned spirit was out there somewhere, crying for a mother.

But later, I would arrive home to see my daughter with new eyes. She seemed more magical, more improbably perfect, than ever before. I watched her, not believing our fortune. Not only was our family healthy and happy, but also, Josephine had come to us first, allowing us the strength to try again, at least one more time.

Within a few days, my body began feeling like my own again. I had a great deal more energy, and I felt motivated to play at a toddler's pace. My abdomen no longer felt tight and tender, and my clothes fit more comfortably. Food tasted better. Smells were no longer nauseating. My dreams returned to the mundane. In the mornings, coffee was a welcome treat. For the first time in two years, I was no longer pregnant or breastfeeding, and I was eager to recover the singular me from the mothering machine my body had become. I could have felt guilty about such a petty pleasure. But my body itself encouraged me, working toward ovulation, doggedly seeking its way back to a regular rhythm. Marvelously single-minded and secure in its purpose, my cycle anchored and comforted me.

On the fourth day after the surgery, I came down with a cold. It was a relief to suffer such a common woe. That evening, with my achy neck and clogged nose, I decided to go to my last yoga class at the elementary school. Leaving Dan and Josephine to their dinner, I took my mat and stepped out into the white, frozen night.

In the warm library, I unrolled my mat, lay down on my back, looked up at the platform ceiling, and overflowed. There we were, the half dozen of us, tucked between shelves displaying Native

American research dioramas, each with a different sixth-grader's hand-lettered DO NOT TOUCH. One thought filled my mind: *I miss you.* I missed the sweet little secret of him. Yoga practice had been our time together—the only time, week in and week out, when I purposefully focused on the pregnancy and strove to connect with the being inside. Yes, some nights at bedtime, I had placed a quiet hand on my abdomen, but those moments carried more worry. I had dedicated my Wednesday yoga classes to simply bonding with my growing fetus, with no judgment, no presentiments, no looking back or ahead. This was the first time I had attended class without him. As I lay on my back, tears slid over my temples and pooled in my ears. As we got moving, my nose ran onto my mat. I had been feeling so good that I was hoping I had been wrong about needing to struggle through three awful crying sessions before I could move on. I had forced the first one into my pillow the day after the results came back. The second had been split in half by the procedure itself. Now, here was the third.

No sooner would I collect myself than the instructor would suggest a new pose for the group: happy baby, final resting pose, fetal position. Each one tore me open afresh. During happy baby, in which we lay on our backs, knees to armpits, feet up, hands grasping the soles, and gently rolling side to side, I realized that for all my worries about sending a tormented soul out into the universe, I had never allowed for the possibility of a happy baby—a soul at peace.

Class ended. I zipped my coat, strapped my boots tight, and, tears still streaming, burst onto the slippery sidewalk. All the way home, three lines kept running through my head: *I miss you. I love you. I will always be your mother.*

epilogue

As I tell you these stories, you are only a dream. You are a comforting presence, a promise somehow alive. You have taken up a place in my heart. Before long, you might take up a place in my womb. We are waiting, if not ready. The methods lay before us, each a glittering, at times terrible, tool. I don't know how, or when, we will meet you. But I still believe we will.

You have not been mapped, charted, or explored. You are not a medal or a prize. You are not our reward. You are not perfection. You are simply a child—our child. An opening has been made for you. You—perhaps a son, perhaps a daughter. You, perhaps a snuggler, perhaps a runner. We know better than to expect particularities, but sometimes I give myself to imagining your sandy hair, your freckles. Hazel eyes like your sister's. A smile like your father's. Dreams like mine.

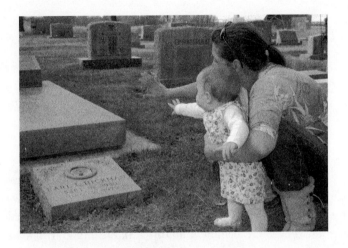

Josephine and Bonnie at Earl's grave in Kimball, Nebraska, 2008

acknowledgments

I owe bottomless thanks to people who shared their stories with me and allowed them to be written. My mother, Paula, was the living storybook and tender heart who inspired this book. For her generosity, openness, and trust in me, my gratitude has no limit. For his part, my brother, Luke, astonished me with his generosity of spirit: Whenever I asked him to judge my fairness, he responded only with encouragement and compassion. My sister, Amanda, shored me up as always, both in writing and in life. My father, Tom, steadfastly imparted to all of our family a sense of security, despite our many unknowns.

For validating my curiosity and giving so much of themselves, I thank my grandmother Esta, my uncles Greg and Curt, my great aunt Sadie, and my cousin Sarah. I am also indebted to Anita Larson, Wilma Costello, Jack Lewis (particularly for photographs and artifacts), Mary Lewis, Joyce Muxlow, Betsy Calhoun, and members of J. R. Gronquist's family.

I am appreciative of the many people who smoothed my access to historical information in Colorado, Wyoming, Nebraska, Washington, and Alberta. They include Weld County sheriff John Cooke; Weld Library district librarian Margaret Langley; Weld County chief deputy coroner Thomas Shimp; former Weld County coroner Paul Stoddard; employees of the cities of Evans and Greeley, Colorado; the Weld County clerk and recorder; Allnut Funeral Service of Greeley; the Colorado Historical Society; the Wyoming Department of State Parks and Cultural Resources; the Barons History Book Club; the organizers of the 2004 Barons Centennial Celebration, especially Mary Bishop; and the records departments of the University of Washington Medical Center and Harborview Medical Center.

Thank you to those doctors and specialists in Ectodermal Dysplasia syndromes whose research and explanations I have used, especially Dr. Virginia Sybert, Dr. Angus J. Clarke, Dr. Olivier Gaide, Dr. Pascal Schneider, and Dr. Robert A. Clark, who was one of my grandfather's best physicians. I am particularly appreciative of the National Foundation for Ectodermal Dysplasias (NFED) for its honest, informed, and loving support of so many families, including my own.

To the various doctors and genetic counselors, named and unnamed in this book, who have expertly and tenderly cared for me, I am profoundly grateful.

My agent, Michelle Brower, saw the significance of this book even in early, messy drafts. I thank her for rolling up her sleeves and helping me find its center. Roxanna Aliaga has my deepest admiration and gratitude for editing my prose with a masterly hand, a gifted mind, and a warm heart. I am thankful to the entire publishing team at Counterpoint for artfully, sensitively, and collaboratively giving physical form to the book I dreamed of.

For their mentorship, I am deeply grateful to Robin Hemley, Patricia A. Foster, David Hamilton, and David Shields. For encouraging me and facilitating my writing process, I thank Maggie McKnight, Jynelle Gracia, Angela Balcita, Alex Sheshunoff, Sarah Kalish Sheshunuff, Jen Rarity, Erin Frerichs, Chrissy Vaughn, Kelly Nakashima, Lara Greden, Shan Nelson, Jessica Peterson, Kate Hopper, and Eula Biss. For their sheer enthusiasm and perfect questions, thank you to Adam and Jenny Gershon.

I am indebted to Dan Jones, editor of the *Modern Love* column of *The New York Times*, as well as the editors of *The Sun* magazine, where the seeds of this book were first published. For their financial support of this project, I am tremendously grateful to the Bush Foundation, the McKnight Foundation, the Minnesota State Arts Board, the Ludwig Vogelstein Foundation, the Bread Loaf Writer's Conference, the Kimmel Harding Nelson Center, the Mary Anderson Center, the Kappa Kappa Gamma Foundation, and the University of Iowa.

I am deeply grateful to my parents-in-law, Jean and Jim Rough, for their bottomless love, insight, and support.

Finally: To Dan, thank you for sharing my journey, steadily believing in me, and giving me the daily comfort of knowing my best friend is near. And to our daughter, Josephine: Thank you for making me smile, especially on the hardest days of my life.